Advance

The Sane Food Solution

To all clinicians and individuals who struggle with overeating, *The Sane Food Solution* is a must-read book by a seasoned food addiction clinician with over 30 years of experience. Unlike typical diet books, this compassionate and readable text serves as a roadmap to escape the torment of overeating and find food recovery and sanity. As an addiction physician, I highly endorse this book; nutritionist Theresa Wright explains the bio-social-spiritual syndrome of food addiction and provides a comprehensive recovery framework: the SMERF plan, encompassing Spirituality, Meetings, Exercise, Rest, and Food Plan. By following this guide, with included exercises and practical tips, you or your client can achieve peace with food, manage your weight, and discover a new life of freedom from food obsession. **—Dr. Vera Tarman**

The Sane Food Solution is a superb amalgam of science and decades of experience written by one of the field's pioneers. The reader will do well to explore the concept of "food addiction" presented by the author and see if the proverbial "shoe fits." Doing so offers the promise of freedom from the tyranny of unending diets and self-recrimination. **—Marty Lerner**, Ph.D. CEO, Milestones In Recovery, Inc.

I am perfectly situated to know that Theresa Wright is unsurpassed in her combination of knowledge, skills, and empathy for food addicts. You may rely on what she conveys in these pages to gain understanding and relief if you struggle with food. —**Michael Prager**, Chairman, Food Addiction Institute

Having known and worked with the author for years, *The Sane Food Solution* is the crown jewel of her work, experience and wisdom. The book addresses everything a person experiencing sugar or ultra-processed food addiction needs to know entering into recovery from this disease! I will want all my clients and students to get this book. —**Esther Helga Gudmundsdottir MSc.**, CFAP, Founder and Director of INFACT (International School for Food Addiction Counseling and Treatment)

The SANE FOOD Solution

Transform Your Relationship with Food and Change Your Life

H. THERESA WRIGHT
MS, RD, LDN

Copyright © 2024 H. Theresa Wright

Visit the author's website at www.sanefood.com.

All rights reserved. No part of this publication may be reproduced, distributed, or transmitted in any form or by any means, including photocopying, recording, or other electronic or mechanical methods, without prior written permission of the publisher, except as permitted by U.S. copyright law. For permission requests, contact author@summitpresspublishers.com.

While the author has made every effort to provide accurate internet addresses at the time of publication, neither the publisher nor author assumes any responsibility for errors, or for changes that occur after publication. Neither the author, nor publisher, is responsible for, and should not be deemed to endorse or recommend, any website other than its own, or any content available on the internet (including without limitation at any website, blog page, information page) that is not created by the author, or publisher.

The advice and strategies contained in this book may not be suitable for your situation. Unique experiences and past performances do not guarantee future results. All referenced testimonials are not intended to be representative of typical results, nor are they a guarantee or promise of any results. Rather, individual successes vary and are due to myriad factors such as effort, knowledge, techniques, timing, and experience.

Printed in the United States of America
First Printing, 2024
ISBN: 979-8-9852063-0-2
Library of Congress Number: 2024921604

Summit Press Publishers
P.O. Box 1356
Intervale, New Hampshire 03845

For information about special discounts available for bulk purchase, workshops, retreats, and webinars associated with this book or offered by H. Theresa Wright, please contact her at www.sanefood.com.

SUMMIT PRESS
PUBLISHERS

This book is dedicated to Jeff Wright,
who has stood beside me through thick and thin.

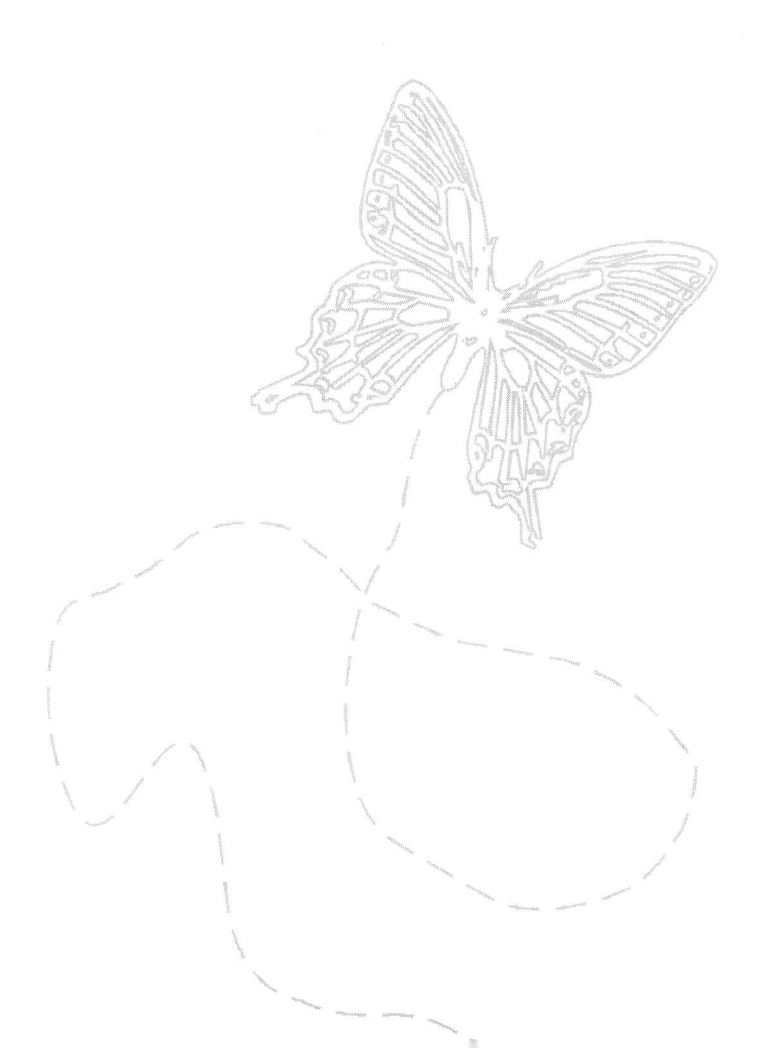

Table of Contents

Introduction ix

Chapter 1: How Does Addiction Work? 1

Chapter 2: Start with How You Think 17

Chapter 3: Embracing Abstinence 31

Chapter 4: Freedom from Trigger, Drug, and Binge Foods 43

Chapter 5: Paving the Way 61

Chapter 6: The Sane Food Eating Plan 71

Chapter 7: Withdrawal, Cravings, and Triggers 89

Chapter 8: Boundaries 111

Chapter 9: Daily Practices 129

Chapter 10: Support Network 149

Chapter 11: Enjoying a New Life 165

A Final Thought 171

Appendix: Withdrawal Symptoms 175

About the Author 179

Introduction

Welcome. You're in the right place. If you have tried many ways of dealing with your problems with food and have not found a solution that works long-term, this book was created to help you.

I'm guessing you may be like many of the people who come to me for help . . .

People like my client, Ardyce: "I'm a creative, well educated, and intelligent woman. I've tried so many diets and weight loss programs: Weight Watchers, NutriSystem, NOOM, South Beach, you name it! . . . They all work, and I lose weight; then something happens, and I'm eating again, and I cannot stop. I tell myself I will start on Monday. Sometimes I will, and sometimes I will not."

Or Patricia: "My husband and I had a huge fight last night. He hates when I try to diet and lose this weight. He says I need more willpower. This morning, I came downstairs to find he had left a box of my favorite doughnuts on the counter, with two removed. I could not decide if I should eat them or stomp on them. Then I'd probably get down on the floor and pick up the crumbs. Instead, I just cried."

Or Jill: "I start a new diet, and for a while I'm just fine. Then, I don't know how it happens. My brain turns off, and I binge the foods I'm missing. When my brain turns back on, I wonder why I did that. It's like I wasn't there and couldn't stop."

Or Karen: "I hate to go to family events where there's food. If I try to follow my plan, I hear, 'Oh, just one piece won't hurt . . . Look how much weight you have lost!' But one bite can lead to a week of bingeing. And if I'm not following the plan, they say, 'Oh, off your plan again, eh?' It hurts. They do not understand the pain I'm suffering."

If you have struggled with food, eating, and body weight for years, you have come to the right place. If you have tried every diet on the planet—from high carb to low or no carb then Paleo—without lasting results, you have come to the right place. If you have gone from fasting to bingeing, if your eating is out of control and you are fed up and frustrated, you have come to the right place. If you just want to learn how to nourish your body well and; if you want to eat in a rational, sane, and healthy way, you have come to the right place.

If you are powerless to control your food intake, resent those who don't understand or fail to support you, are sick and tired of the roller coaster and want nothing more than to give up and curl in on yourself with a pint or three of ice cream, welcome to what this book has to offer.

For the last thirty-seven years I have helped people break free of the compulsion to abuse themselves with food. This is now being called food addiction. While there is a lot of new and exciting information coming out about refined and ultra-processed foods, this disorder combines our sensitivities to such foods with other issues in our lives, which makes it very powerful.

Jill and Patricia (and many of the others I work with) have a physical sensitivity to certain foods. This sensitivity has been named lots of things, but it really means that your body has changed in a significant way. It's an addition; we may hate the word because of its ties to heroin and other illicit substances, but that's what it is. Food addiction is an umbrella term meaning a physical change has happened with certain foods.

INTRODUCTION

Americans—my clients included—face a major struggle with food, eating, body weight, and a host of horrifying diseases like diabetes, heart disease, and hypertension. As a society, sixty to eighty percent of us are overweight or obese. Weight loss diets abound, and we go on and off them with abandon. These diets all work for a bit, but the weight invariably comes back, along with a ton of shame. No doubt, you can attest to this as well.

But here's the thing: until you find and solve the underlying problem, the battle with food and the scale will keep you in a chokehold. You can yo-yo diet all you want; the problem will return.

Think about it. If you go to your doctor with an ear infection and he gives you a decongestant and a pain reliever, you will feel better right away, yet only temporarily. Unfortunately, the problem (an ear infection) will remain until you deal with the root cause (a bacterial disturbance) with an antibiotic. Solve the actual problem and the symptoms go away for good.

Similarly, obesity is often the symptom or the result of some other problem or group of problems. Until you find and resolve the other problems, obesity will respond to diets, but quickly return.

That's why, to permanently free yourselves from the pain (and shame) of obesity, which is the number one symptom with which Americans struggle, you must go after the root cause—food addiction. Other things may also play a part, but an eating program that doesn't illuminate addictive substances may not provide true relief.

Food addiction is a physical, genetically inherited biochemical glitch in the way the body handles carbohydrates. (Yes, you can also be sensitive to fats and salts and crunchy or creamy foods—even the need for more!)

If you are a food addict, you handle foods differently than others. First, your brain chemistry has been altered by allergens you've ingested. Scientists don't know why; you're simply susceptible. Your body handles differently all the processed, refined, ultra-processed, and man-made foods that stock our shelves these days. These food stuffs are hard to avoid, and they are harming you. They make the manufacturers oodles of money and make your situation worse; they make your addiction worse. You will never break free of your food obsession until you eliminate these allergens from your diet, until you practice abstinence.

This book is all about helping you do that: find and eliminate the foods you can't eat because they throw your brain chemistry off. Your addiction to these substances is what's keeping you caught in an endless loop of consumption, malaise, and suppression. And it is preventing you from solving the real problems.

I Understand Addiction

I not only understand addiction and the associated chaos from a professional level, I grew up with this stuff. Raised in a tiny town in northeastern Pennsylvania, ten blocks long and four blocks wide, my Daddy was a coal miner. Today my family might be called dysfunctional, alcoholic, abusive, codependent, and other similar names. Back then, it seemed normal.

When I was in eighth grade, they called my dad down to the school and asked if I might go to college. At that time, only boys went to college. Daddy was delighted. He told me I needed to go to a better school than the ones in my area, work hard and get good grades, and make a decent life for myself.

I picked Drexel University, right in the middle of Philadelphia, the "City of Brotherly Love." And I'll never forget my first nutrition class, sitting in that big auditorium, finding myself gob-smacked. I waved my hand at the professor to get his attention and said, "Wait! Stop!

INTRODUCTION

Are you telling me that the chicken I ate for dinner last night is going to become my heart or lungs, or liver or eyeballs?"

"Yes, my dear, that's exactly what I am telling you." He replied. "And I am going to teach you how the body does that."

From that moment on, I was fascinated with the way the body works—how it takes the food we eat and uses it to repair, replace, and maintain itself, clear diseases out of the body, and do all we ask of it with little complaint. How the body digests, absorbs, and metabolizes food and uses it to build the next iteration of ourselves.

That's terrific news if you're overweight, obese, or have a whole host of medical problems. You may have run the whole gamut of dieting, starving, bingeing, purging, and feeling guilty and awful. You may have tried every new diet program, then "given in" to your desires and regained the lost weight, and then some. You may suffer from mental obsessions about food, eating, and body weight . . . but your body and mind can be changed with the right help. You can become someone else. It's fascinating, and the reason I've been obsessed with these ideas for nearly sixty years.

In our society, we do not regard food and eating as the miracle maker it could be. We regard our food and eating behaviors as right or wrong, good or bad, healthy or not. We indulge in many food and eating behaviors that are not designed to nourish or support the body. When we gain weight, we simply look to one of the many diets that abound to force the body to release the unacceptable pounds. I think of a diet as the period of deprivation that happens right before you gain twenty pounds or more.

Food, it seems, has become our enemy.

In reality, the right food in the right quantities can be your salvation. Food can be the key to your mental health and your physical transformation.

Obesity and eating disorders are the symptom, the cause, or the result of another problem or group of problems. Once you solve the problems, peace of mind and heart, a normal body weight, neutrality with food, and a joyful, useful life of our dreams are possible. Changing your food choices to those that support and nourish the body, to those that enhance your well-being, will lead to the ability to solve the problems in your life, maintain the health and well-being of your body, and transform yourself into the person you have always wanted to become.

Helping you do that is the purpose of this book. (I've also created additional training and resources on my site, which you can access here: www.sanefood.com/bonus.)

Together, we'll look at the chaos around food, eating, and body weight and consider your food choices and the impact they have on your body, mind, and spirit. It starts by making sane choices.

The Sane Food Solution

Wikipedia defines sanity as, "the soundness, rationality, and health of the human mind, as opposed to insanity." G.K. Chesterton states, sanity involves wholeness, whereas insanity implies narrowness and brokenness.[1]

So, according to these definitions, if you have lost your ability to think and behave in a rational manner, you're broken. That's why many twelve-step programs have their members recite a line that describes a major turning point in their recovery process: "Came to believe that a Power greater than ourselves could restore us to sanity."

---

[1] Dale Ahlquist, "Lecture 4: Robert Browning," Chesterton University, June 15, 2024. http://www.chesterton.org/lecture-4.

INTRODUCTION

Food itself is neither sane nor insane, good nor bad. But the way we choose and use food can be sane or insane. It can be reasonable and rational, or chaotic and abusive. If you can relate, if you feel you are no longer in control when it comes to food, there is hope.

I created the Sane Food Solution as a way of discussing a return to healthy eating. It is the consumption of whole food, real food, processed as little as possible. It does not include "man-made foods" or "edible food-like objects." It meets the body's nutrient needs; it takes the body to a normal weight and encourages health and well-being. It improves your ability to think clearly, make good decisions, and grow into the person you want to become.

Sane food behaviors are:

- **S**ustainable
- **A**bundant
- **N**utrient-rich
- **E**ffective at meeting your goals
- **F**ree of binge, drug, and trigger foods
- **O**pen to change and adaptation
- **O**ptimal for your recovery
- **D**elicious

By contrast, insane food behaviors cause you to bounce up and down by twenty pounds without knowing why. They make you afraid of the scale; prevent your slacks from zipping. They stir up feelings of blame, guilt, sorrow, shame, and self-hatred. They make you feel completely out of control, hungry all the time, or stuffed at one meal and starving at another. Insane food behaviors trigger your cravings and increase your feelings of discomfort or self-dislike. They increase your addictive and compulsive behaviors, and whenever you stop using them, you experience withdrawal symptoms.

The Sane Food Solution is the middle ground. It's not dieting, bingeing, starving, or stuffing; it's not beating the body or abusing the spirit. It's about practicing kindness, self-respect, and gratitude. It involves meeting the body's nutrient needs and the spirit's emotional needs without struggle, compulsion, cravings, self-abuse, or self-hatred. (If you're curious, we'll discuss these principles in detail in Chapter 7.)

When you replace insane food behaviors with sane food behaviors, you will finally be relaxed and comfortable with food and eating. You'll have few cravings and generally feel satisfied. Your body will be healthy and energetic. You will also feel your feelings and know how to appropriately handle them. You will learn to lean on others for help and grow into your life and your recovery program.

The Recovery Process

The Sane Food Solution is not a quick fix. It's a recovery process, one that you can maintain long-term and is not harmful to its environment—mainly you. This process involves several key components.

When it comes time to create your food plan, it needs to be individualized; it needs to consider your age, height, weight, lifestyle, food preferences, and medical conditions. It needs to fit your body like the perfect pair of sneakers fit your feet: supportive, protective, comfortable, and well able to carry you safely over rough ground.

Following your plan may be hard at first because change is tough and lots of chaos arises. For one, you'll not be eating the standard American fare—and it's hard to be out in the world, eating differently from everyone else. Until you settle into this new way of eating, you may feel left out of the fun. As a society, we enjoy food to celebrate a birth, a birthday, a religious passage, a wedding, another birth, and to grieve the death of a loved one. When you change the way you participate, you may begin to question your choices, and so will others.

Celebrations and grief are not the only ways food is used in expression of our lives; it may be used to create friendships, express our ethnicity and moral preferences—it may even help us manage our anxiety and sorrow. If you experience major problems with food, eating, and body weight, food serves many more purposes. When it's no longer an option, you'll need to find other ways to satisfy those needs.

As a result, you'll likely experience physical withdrawal: anxiety, irritability, and anger. If you've been avoiding past traumas and feelings or stuffing them down with food, they'll come flying up in vivid detail.

But I'm going to show you how to deal with all of this and more.

Like my professor taught me all those years ago, nutrient-rich food will change your brain cells and every other cell in your body. When you know what your body (and lifestyle) needs, you'll be able to manage the grocery store, your employer's dinner party, your mother-in-law's visit, and the challenges you'll face simply because you're alive and human.

Your efforts will be rewarded with incredible peace and freedom. You will be able to walk through your days with joy and purpose. You will feel healthy and strong and create the life you have always wanted.

You will stand with the *Big Book of Alcoholics Anonymous* and say, "We have ceased fighting anything or anyone. We feel as though we had been placed in a position of neutrality—safe and protected."[2] This is my wish for you.

---

[2] *Alcoholics Anonymous Big Book.* (New York: Alcoholics Anonymous World Services, 2002), 84–85.

Chapter 1

How Does Addiction Work?

Food can change your brain cells, and that changes your thinking and your behavior. That's because certain chemicals found in the brain, stomach, and bloodstream make you respond in certain ways. They're called neurotransmitters, and they're deeply involved in the physical process of addiction.

Just as birds fly, fish swim, and drunks drink, food addicts eat. To want to eat everything that's not nailed down and does not bite back is as normal to a food addict as breathing, so are cravings. The impulse to go back to old behaviors, no matter how well or how long you have stuck to sane eating, never really goes away. Such behaviors and impulses are all signs of a physical sensitivity to something in the food, even if you haven't eaten that food in a while.

Your body, mind, and spirit react differently to refined and over-processed foods. That's all there is to it. That physical change is called an addiction. Before long, you don't simply react physically to these substances, you begin to see food as a comfort, a reward—as your sanity. Food becomes your all. Take that food out of your diet, and the body, mind, and spirit will constantly call you back. The call may be insistent to the point of demanding, compulsive, or irresistible.

In the groups I lead, people often share some variant of this statement: "I've been struggling with food for decades; some days I'm willing to follow my food plan, and some days I just don't care. I feel that I *need* the food to get through the day."

One of the criteria for addiction is compulsion: the inability to stop; loss of control; continued use despite harmful consequences; and physical withdrawal symptoms. But addiction often also includes a psychological need to change one's feelings over and above the physical constructs of demand and distress or withdrawal.

Drugs like food, sex, gambling, alcohol, and sugar give prompt, effective short-term relief and pleasure, then euphoria, followed by an emotional low that frequently encourages re-use. Acquisition becomes important; the person needs more to relieve physical discomfort.

After a four-year process involving more than eighty experts, the American Society of Addiction Medicine recently released a new definition of addiction: "At its core, addiction isn't just a social problem or a moral problem or a criminal problem. It's a brain problem whose behaviors manifest in all these other areas." Dr. Michael Miller, past president of the American Society of Addiction Medicine, who oversaw the development of the new definition, said, "Many behaviors driven by addiction are real problems and sometimes criminal acts. But the disease is about brains, not drugs; it's about underlying neurology, not outward actions." The new definition also describes addiction as a primary disease, meaning it's not the result of other causes, such as emotional or psychiatric problems. Like cardiovascular disease and diabetes, addiction is recognized as a chronic disease; therefore, it must be treated, managed, and monitored over a person's lifetime.

> **At its core, addiction isn't just a social problem or a moral problem or a criminal problem. It's a brain problem whose behaviors manifest in all these other areas.**

So, food addiction is not about moral depravity or lack of willpower or, of fear or failure (though seductive advertising may sway us to believe this is the case). Compulsion is a symptom of physical withdrawal and the accompanying change in your neurotransmitters. You're at a disadvantage if you don't see that because it decreases your sense of personal responsibility, trapping you in behavior patterns inconsistent with conscious thought or will. Once you see compulsion for what it is, you can take back your power.

Plain and Simple

The whole point of eating is to give your body the nutrients it needs to repair, replace, and maintain itself. When you eat primarily processed and low-nutrient foods, foods with many added substances, the body can do little with the chemicals other than store them. When you eat foods with lots of sugar and other processed chemicals, it causes the changes in the functioning of your brain cells to accelerate.

Apart from glucose, which is a natural substance in the body, even the tiniest amounts of substances that are foreign to the body can cause a reaction. They do that by releasing neurotransmitters in your brain that change and smooth out your feelings. It's a physical force inside your body, mind, and spirit that makes you focus on wanting more and getting more . . . and more.

If your body wants more of what it's used to and you feel as though you cannot live without those foods, this is addiction.

If you have intense and powerful cravings, a feeling of desperation when they're not available, and thoughts that focus only on when and how you can get more, this is addiction.

If you can relate to this compulsion, then you're likely an addict. So, freeing yourself from food's tight grip will involve changing the way you eat, abstaining from key substances, managing your emotions, and developing strategic responses to temptations.

Before we get to the food part, let's address the heart of the problem—your thoughts.

For now, we're going to examine the physical changes that happen in everyone's brain when they eat certain foods. Then we'll move into how the food addict's brain responds, which differs from that of the non-addict.

For those of you who want to know the specific details of this process, please keep reading. If you're not interested in such details, you can simply skip the rest of this chapter and go on to the next chapter.

How the Brain Works

The brain is the most complex entity in the universe. It is an enormous switchbox housing trillions of interconnected pathways, containing about fifty billion cells called neurons, with trillions of interconnections among the neurons. Neurons are the switches that control the flow of information carried by neurotransmitters, which are chemical messengers that control emotions, perceptions, and bodily functions. A complicated relationship among thought, feeling, and brain chemistry exists because of the way the brain communicates with the rest of the body, which is why we need to understand the interconnectedness when addressing addiction.

Networks of neurons send signals back and forth—to each other and among different parts of the brain, the spinal cord, and nerves in the rest of the body (the peripheral nervous system). To send a message, a neuron releases a chemical neurotransmitter into the gap (or synapse) between it and the next cell. The neurotransmitter crosses the synapse and attaches to receptors on the receiving neuron, like a key into a lock, which causes changes in the receiving cell. Other molecules (called transporters) recycle neurotransmitters . . . they bring them back into the neuron that released them, thereby limiting or shutting off the signal between neurons. In some cases, shutting off a signal is a good thing; in other cases, shutting off a signal wreaks havoc.

How Addictive Substances Change the Brain

The neuron has three basic parts. There is a central nucleus called the soma and two long, sweeping "legs"—the dendron and the axon. The dendron receives messages from the neurons; the axon transmits messages to the neurons; and the soma decides whether to send a message through the axon to neighboring neurons. We call this firing. The intensity of the fired signal comes from the frequency of firing and the total amount of neurotransmitter released.

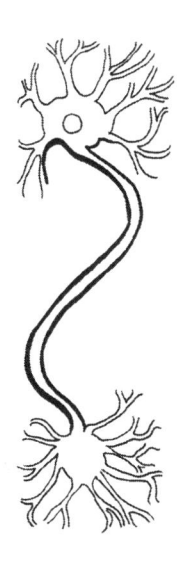

This is the axon tube. One end receives messages; they are transmitted to the other end of the tube, where they are released. This is how messages travel in the brain.

When the soma receives a message from its dendron and decides to fire, a chemical neurotransmitter is released into the intracellular fluid between the neurons.

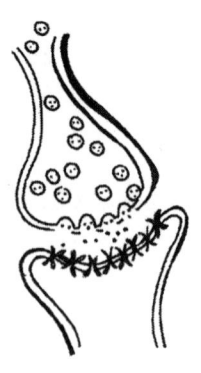

The axon holds the messengers called neurotransmitters and releases them into the fluid between itself and the next axon.

As it floats, it is picked up by the receptors on the next neuron, and the message is transmitted.

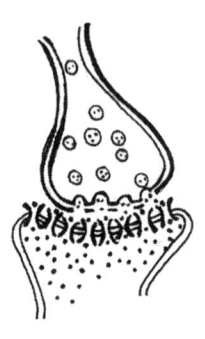

Receptor sites on the next axon pick up the transmitters and carry the message.

When sensitivities come into play, the neurons release more neurotransmitter than normal, causing the neighboring neurons to make more receptors.

But a neurotransmitter is not easily fooled. Anytime you give a food or drug to increase the amount of a neurotransmitter, the synapse will remove receptors for that neurotransmitter, effectively making itself less sensitive to that drug. This process is known as down-regulation. Conversely, if you try to decrease the amount of a neurotransmitter present, the synapse will try to make itself more sensitive by recruiting more receptors to the cell surface, known as up-regulation. These processes account for much of what is observed during drug tolerance and withdrawal.

Euphoria Surges and the Addict's Brain

In some people, sugar and highly processed foods interfere with the way neurons send, receive, and process signals. The exact mechanism of this interference is not fully known, but it's similar to that caused by drugs like heroin or cocaine.

Pleasure or euphoria—the high from sugar and highly processed foods—is still poorly understood. It was once thought that surges of the neurotransmitter dopamine produced by drugs directly caused the euphoria, but scientists now think dopamine has more to do with getting us to repeat pleasurable activities (reinforcement) than with producing pleasure directly.

In other words, it probably involves surges of chemical signaling compounds, including the body's natural opioids (endorphins) and other neurotransmitters in the reward circuit part of the brain. When these food substances are eaten, they can cause surges of these neurotransmitters much greater than the smaller bursts naturally produced in association with healthy rewards like eating, hearing or playing music, creative pursuits, or social interaction.

The feeling of pleasure is how a healthy brain identifies and reinforces beneficial behaviors, such as eating, socializing, and sex. Our brains are wired to increase the odds that we will repeat pleasurable activities. The neurotransmitter dopamine is central to this. Whenever the reward circuit is activated by a healthy, pleasurable experience, a burst of dopamine signals that something important is happening that needs to be remembered. This dopamine signal causes changes in neural connectivity that make it easier to repeat the activity again and again without thinking about it, leading to the formation of habits.

Just as sugar and highly processed foods can produce intense euphoria, they also produce much larger surges of dopamine, powerfully reinforcing the connection between consumption of the drug, the resulting pleasure, and all the external cues linked to the experience. Large surges of dopamine "teach" the brain to seek these foods at the expense of other, healthier goals and activities.

Cues in a person's daily routine or environment that have become linked with certain foods can trigger uncontrollable cravings whenever the person is exposed to the cues, even if the foods are not available. This learned "reflex" can last a long time. For example, people who have been abstinent for a decade can experience cravings when returning to an old neighborhood or house where they ate those foods. Like riding a bike, the brain remembers.

And the brain adjusts. Just as we turn down the volume on a radio that's too loud, the brain of someone who misuses food adjusts. Specifically, there is an intricate system of modulation and control in the transmission of impulses in the brain. When larger amounts are consumed, the brain tries to adjust to keep everything "normal," and the receptors start to shut down. This is a physical change in the neurons, and the message of pleasure is reduced.

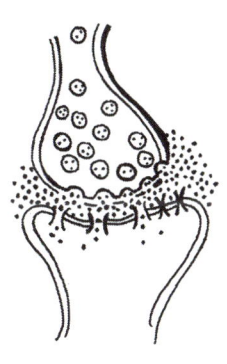

If you eat too much of a given food, the receptors get overwhelmed and shut off. This is the process of addiction; the receptors are overwhelmed and shut off, so you do not get the good feelings from the food (or other drug).

As a result, the person's ability to experience pleasure from naturally rewarding activities is also reduced. The person needs to eat more and more of the food to experience even a normal level of reward (an effect known as tolerance)—which only makes the problem worse. It's a vicious cycle.

This is why those who misuse food eventually feel flat, lifeless, depressed, without motivation, and unable to enjoy things that were previously pleasurable.

The start of the addictive process feels so good! Yet, at some point there was a physical change in the structure of the neurons in the brain, which caused a change in the neurochemical reactions. Therefore, food addiction is not a value judgment. You did nothing wrong; you are not a bad person—we're not talking about street drugs here. It simply means a physical change has happened in your brain and you are physically sensitive to certain food, and now you must learn to live with that reality.

Repairing Your Brain

Addictive substances actually change the structure of the brain. They may change the regulation of a membrane or make it stiffer or softer. The chemicals allowed inside the cell may change and impair cell function. The receptors may change. They may require more or less of the substance; they may stiffen and not respond. You may need a much higher dose to achieve the same effect, or you may get no effect at all. These changes in brain chemicals may change your mood—up, down, or sideways. They can alter your thinking, your behavior, and your decision-making.

It's important to know that you can change brain chemistry by changing your behavior. It may take a long time; it could take six months to a year (or more) before your brain and reward systems begin to heal. Unfortunately, they may not seem to go back to their original levels; the addictive changes and intolerances persist long-term.

> **It's important to know that you can change brain chemistry by changing your behavior.**

When you stop eating the foods to which you're sensitive, withdrawal symptoms will appear. They may last anywhere from thirty days to a year. In withdrawal, many strange symptoms crop up: heightened sensitivity, impaired judgement, overreaction to stress, and food thoughts or cues. Cravings can become intense. These symptoms confirm the physical change of addiction.

To address the chemical imbalance that rules your thoughts, feelings, and behaviors, you need to pay attention to key neurotransmitters and their role in your brain and your recovery.

Neurotransmitters of Addiction

There are forty different neurotransmitters created in the body, each with its own purpose. How you feel and how you think are determined by which neurotransmitters are released into which synapses. So, let's look at the neurotransmitters of addiction; here are the most closely related to food and their functions.

Acetylcholine (ACH) helps us remember things and process information. It is the neurotransmitter that functions at the voluntary and involuntary nerve-muscle connections and nerve-system synapses. Choline, which is converted into acetylcholine, is found in many foods, including beef liver (or top round), eggs, roasted chicken, cod, soybeans, kidney beans, cooked quinoa, mushrooms, broccoli, and Brussels sprouts. Isn't that a strange mixture?

When a food addict consumes a high-sugar diet, their insulin production increases abruptly. Protein—and choline-producing foods—will normalize insulin to stabilize blood sugar. It also stabilizes your mood. So, you must be sure that you are getting enough protein.

Glutamate is the most abundant excitatory (causing excitation, or energy) neurotransmitter in your brain and central nervous system. It's needed to keep your brain functioning properly. Glutamate plays a major role in learning and memory. Also, glutamate helps regulate your sleep/awake cycle.

Many foods block glutamate, which leads to impulsivity and anger, as well as difficulty finding new coping mechanisms. You may have more physical and emotional pain. Problems from the past may resurrect themselves to torture you. That is how difficult feelings return again and again.

The goal of The Sane Food Solution is to take those glutamate-blocking foods like sugar out of your system to better regulate your emotions.

Dopamine has been labeled the "feel-good chemical" because of its role in our satiety, pleasure, mood, and desires. Dopamine is the neurotransmitter released for reward and motivation. This is the brain's way of rewarding us for engaging in basic life-sustaining behaviors such as eating and sex. It gives us pleasure.

It serves as a major transmitter in the part of the brain regulating motor behavior. It enhances learning, regulates emotion and motivation, and appears to be the common neurotransmitter related to food and eating issues.

Eating refined, processed, or man-made food causes a release of dopamine in the brain, encouraging us to eat more of these foods. A healthy meal also can stimulate the release of dopamine; and dopamine may be released in the brain both when the food is first eaten, and when the food has reached the stomach.

The goal of The Sane Food Solution is to eliminate dopamine surges brought about by addictive food, the type that deadens life-sustaining pleasures, so your emotional life isn't held captive by these substances.

Serotonin is our major feel-good, enjoy-life neurotransmitter, and it stabilizes our mood, feelings of well-being, and happiness. Serotonin can be released by laughter, prayer and meditation, exercise, or effective sex. The various functions of serotonin in the central nervous system include sleep, hunger, mood, memory, and learning management. Serotonin creates a long-lasting feeling of happiness or well-being. It enables brain cells and other nervous system cells to communicate with each other.

Low levels of serotonin in the brain may cause depression, anxiety, and sleep trouble. A serotonin deficiency is thought to be associated with several psychological symptoms, such as anxiety, irritability, depressed moods, memory skills, and learning abilities. Medications to treat depression (Selective Serotonin Reuptake Inhibitors) focus on increasing serotonin levels in the brain.

Although serotonin is a well-known brain neurotransmitter, it is estimated that ninety-five percent of the body's serotonin is made in the digestive tract by gut bacteria. Sugar causes serotonin to be released in your brain, which is why the consumption feels so pleasurable. Serotonin is made from the amino acid tryptophan, so high-tryptophan foods will help the body create more serotonin. Foods that contain tryptophan include chicken, turkey, salmon, milk, eggs, spinach, seeds, and most soy products.

The goal of The Sane Food Solution is to replace addictive serotonin boosters—both foods and activities—with a healthier variety, one that won't hijack your mood and ability to process whatever is going on in your life.

Gamma Amino-Butyric Acid (GABA) calms us and relaxes us. GABA also reduces the firing of neurons and slows down neurotransmission. It is very active in the brain synapses; in fact, it may be the predominant neurotransmitter of the brain. It is the transmitter at twenty-five to forty percent of all synapses in the brain. GABA promotes feelings of calm and tiredness by blocking excess dopamine and noradrenaline from overstimulating the brain; this helps to slow down the heart rate and breathing and allows relaxation. GABA is inhibitory, meaning it can help break the anxiety of an overtaxed and overactive mind.

GABA can be synthesized in the intestinal tract by beneficial bacteria. Eating fermented foods that are rich in probiotics, such as sauerkraut, kimchi, miso, tempeh, yogurt, and kefir, can help increase GABA levels. Glutamic acid helps create GABA in the brain. So, it's important to consume foods rich in glutamic acid, including citrus fruits and bananas, almonds, walnuts, spinach, potatoes, broccoli, and lentils.

The goal of The Sane Food Solution is to increase foods that boost GABA production to reduce anxiety and overthinking.

Endorphins make us feel better when we exercise, fall in love, or need our pain reduced. They are not neurotransmitters; they are a group of peptides created by the pituitary gland and hypothalamus. They act on the opiate receptors in your brain to increase feelings of pleasure and well-being and to reduce pain and discomfort. Secretion of endorphins leads to feelings of euphoria, changes of appetite, and increased immune response. With high endorphin levels, one feels less pain and less stress.

Endorphins can be released by a massage, hot bath, laughter, music, dancing, meditation, effective sex, a random act of kindness, or fifteen minutes of sunshine. (Sure, chocolate, wine, and other high-fat foods can do this, but they are not consistent with our goals.)

Foods that release endorphins include avocados, chilis, hot peppers, legumes and nuts, asparagus, oranges, broccoli, and peppers.

The goal of The Sane Food Solution is to replace suboptimal foods with optimal foods for feelings of pleasure and to release endorphins through life-affirming activities.

The Goals

When it comes to your recovery food program, you want enough protein so that your insulin can stay stable; you want to take addictive and overprocessed foods out of your system to better regulate your emotions. You want to enhance learning, regulate emotions, and replace addictive foods and activities with healthier options that won't hijack your mood and ability to process.

You want to reduce anxiety and worry and enjoy the pleasures of your new recovering life. And since a major purpose of food is to provide the nutrients the body needs to repair, replace, and maintain itself, let's go for a healthy body too.

So, you may be asking, "Food and recovery activities can do that?" Yes, indeed. Let me show you how . . .

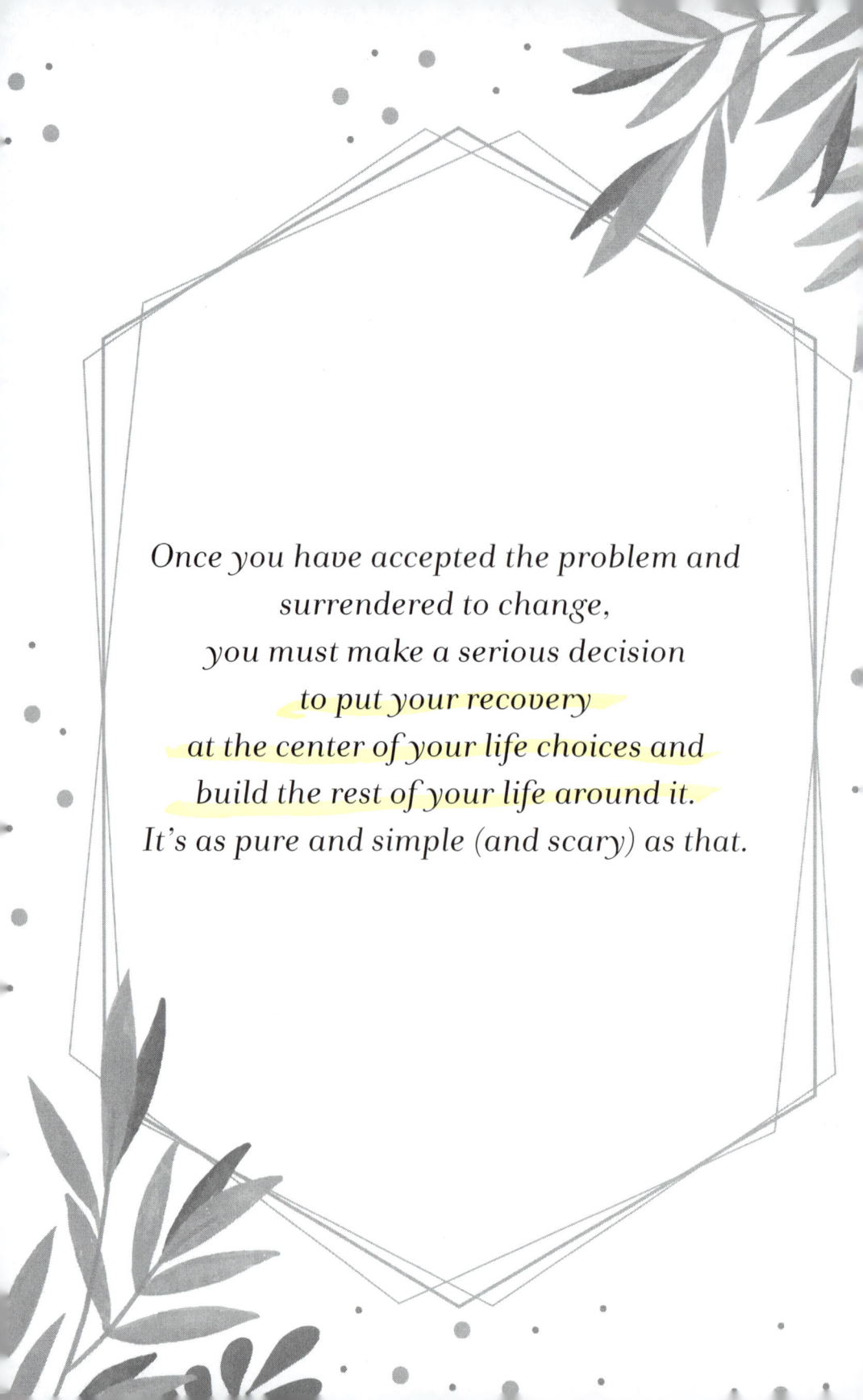

Once you have accepted the problem and
surrendered to change,
you must make a serious decision
to put your recovery
at the center of your life choices and
build the rest of your life around it.
It's as pure and simple (and scary) as that.

Chapter 2
Start with How You Think

You've struggled with food, eating, and body weight issues for a long time. Maybe it started when you were little: your mom gave you cookies any time you were hurt, Halloween candy held no boundaries, you stole money from purses to buy candy. Maybe you took your weekly allowance to the grocery store and bought as much candy as you could, then hid somewhere to eat it all in peace. Maybe food was a reward for some kind of abuse. Maybe food was the response *to* abuse, the thing that got you through it.

If this is you, you are certainly not alone. Over the last thirty years of helping obese (overweight, underweight, struggling) people free themselves from their food addiction, I estimate fifty to seventy percent of them were running from some kind of unhealthy, frightening, or abusive childhood experiences. Not all, but most.

As these brave people have taught me, recovery starts with your thoughts. To treat your body with dignity and respect, to nourish it back to health, you need to retrain your mind. You need to develop a strategic response to temptation. You need to learn how to release your feelings of deprivation and reach for peace and freedom. You need to challenge your addictive thinking, banish thoughts that hold you down, and replace them with positive thoughts to recreate your world.

How to Help Your Brain Cope

Abstinence is difficult. Removing addictive substances from your diet permanently in order to heal your brain will bring up the feelings you used food to suppress. In order to move forward, you will need to do four things:

1. **Grieve**. In many ways, the foods to which you are sensitive have become your partner, best friend, or primary supporter down through the years. You may not know what to do with your time, with your evenings, with your hands. Allow yourself some time to feel sad, empty, alone, at loose ends. The key is not to wallow in those feelings.

2. **Learn new skills**. A lot of things will change. To start, you'll need to learn a new way to select, acquire, and prepare your food. If your social life was built around eating and body weight, you'll need to discover new ways of interacting with others. If it doesn't come naturally, learn to see the fun in learning something new.

3. **Face the reasons you were eating**. Food worked better for you than anything else to make the pain stop. When you no longer "medicate" the pain away, feelings, problems, memories of unresolved issues may resurface.

4. **Don't try to bargain your way around it**. You know how it goes, telling yourself, *Diets work, if only you stay on them . . . that person can eat the food I love and maintain a*

healthy weight, surely I can too. Don't ignore the real issue by keeping yourself busy or trying yet another weight loss program. It won't work. If you attend an Overeaters Anonymous meeting because, you know, *I may be on to something,* the minute you hear, "Give up sugar," you'll quit.

For lasting change, you must face the real reason behind your addiction, which means you must recognize (and address) your feelings of denial and powerlessness, so you can accept the issue, surrender to change, and ultimately set yourself up for a new way of thinking. For a very long time, you've used food to manage your feelings. Once you stop abusing food, you will need to manage these feelings in a healthier way.

Denial

Maybe you're thinking, *Got it; just give me the Sane Food Plan, and I'll be on my merry way.* But you're not ready for that yet. There is one more word we haven't talked about. It has a few spellings: DeNile; The Nile . . . Denial. It's not a river in Egypt. It's a river in your life that you refuse to see.

Denial is an important component of addiction. It allows addiction to run the show uninterrupted. And in the course of my work as a dietitian, I see denial every single day: the fellow who says, "If only my boss would behave differently," the woman who proclaims, "I don't intend to live my life without my favorite foods. That's Ridiculous!"

These people refuse to see the truth about themselves, their lives, and their relationships with other people or with food. They refuse! This is denial.

The concept of denial arose from the work of Sigmund Freud, whose daughter, Anna Freud, developed the idea of defense mechanisms: unconscious strategies whereby people protect themselves from anxious thoughts or feelings. Anna believed that denial unconsciously protects the ego from discomfort and distress by rejecting certain aspects of reality; if employed regularly into adulthood, it could be damaging.

Although many of Freud's ideas have been disproven, psychologists today still believe that defense mechanisms are a valid concept—and that denial does, indeed, cause harm because it prevents you from taking action to deal with the problem.[1]

If you are in denial, you are trying to protect yourself from a truth too painful for you to accept at the moment. Sometimes short-term denial is essential. It can give you time to organize yourself and accept a significant change in your life. However, denial can have a darker side and become unhealthy.

People deny they have an addictive problem with food or that food addiction even exists. No one wants to consider themselves an addict. If they continue to function and go to work each day, they tend to not consider the amount of time, energy, money, and mental and emotional energy they are spending regularly on unhealthy foods.

The Four Kinds of Denial

There are four kinds of denial:

1. **Denial of fact**—when you refuse to acknowledge that the problem is a real one. This is the first level and a real challenge.

[1.] Psychology Today, "Denial," accessed August 25, 2024, https://www.psychologytoday.com/us/basics/denial.

2. **Denial of impact**—when you minimize the importance of the problem. "I have to stop eating sugar; lots of people have diabetes." The answer is to not only admit that the food and eating problem exists, but that it's having a serious effect on your quality of life and keeping you from having the things you really want.

3. **Denial of responsibility**—when you attempt to avoid responsibility by explaining that your actions and circumstances are somehow out of your control. This is where you'll hear, "I was stressed out; the cravings were overwhelming; I just couldn't stop."

4. **Denial of hope**—when you refuse to acknowledge the real problem and are unwilling to do the work needed to improve the situation. "I don't want to live the rest of my life without sugar; I hate being different from everyone else; people will think I'm strange; I won't be part of the group." Such statements are a game stopper because they indicate you are unwilling to take the steps needed to make things better.

How to Spot Denial

Perhaps you are in denial about your denial. That is, after all, what it's all about: fooling yourself regarding the reality of your situation.

You are in denial if you:

- Avoid talking about the real problem.
- Talk endlessly about the symptoms that annoy you.
- Avoid letting others help you.

- Find ways to justify your behavior.
- Blame other people or outside forces for causing the problem.
- Persist in a behavior despite negative consequences.
- Avoid thinking about the problem or complain about it without considering the solution.
- Promise to address the problem in the future.

Denial is insidious; it creeps in, drop by drop. You may not notice it at first, but before long, precious parts of your life begin to rot or melt away. The only way to stop it is to open your eyes and confront it—to make changes quickly, before you're badly hurt. And while there may be a lot of ways to engage in denial, there's only one way to fully accept responsibility: do the work.

And it takes emotional strength. Which is why you must overcome any feelings of powerlessness.

Powerlessness

Hard as this is to believe, you are not the most powerful force in the universe. You need only look at how you stack up against the forces of nature to see that's true. In a way, addiction is its own force of nature—one that requires a particular kind of help to overcome being powerless.

"Wait, what do you mean, I'm powerless . . . powerless over Twinkies and Ding-Dongs? Please. I'm strong in every other area of my life. I have a good job; I own my own home. I'd be entirely happy if I could just lose weight!"

START WITH HOW YOU THINK

Yet, if you ask why they can't lose weight (or keep it off, which is worse), they have no answer. I've heard it many times before, one client after another. They've lost the weight twenty times; it's keeping it off—dealing with the cravings and compulsions—that keep sending them back to the food. They give no specifics; they don't really know; they simply can't. They're powerless.

Being powerless over food does not mean you can't stop eating all foods, only some foods. Usually, they are foods specific to you. Powerlessness means there is a point at which you cannot stop, even if you want to. It means that, unaided, you are unable to accomplish your goal, that the outcome is not in your control.

Powerlessness is not weakness or laziness; it's not immoral. If you could have accomplished this by yourself, you would have done so already. Don't demean yourself; it will further diminish your power and sense of self.

> **Powerlessness is not weakness or laziness; it's not immoral. If you could have accomplished this by yourself, you would have done so already.**

There are many benefits to recognizing your powerlessness; it:

(1) Gives you back your power. It may seem a strange juxtaposition, but it's true. When you admit you are powerless and stop fighting the food, you can begin to feel the pain and process the feelings—and that is how you access the power to change your life. It's not available to you when you are using it to battle Twinkies and Ding Dongs.

(2) Gives you the chance to know yourself more intimately. You'll be able to come into touch with your "inner core of wisdom," or, as Deepak Chopra says, "the ageless, timeless eternal you," in a new and different way. You get the

chance to change yourself into the person you want to become.

(3) Gets you in touch with a spiritual power—at least, it gives you a good excuse to search it out. Finding a power greater than you allows you to grow and solve problems more effectively.

(4) Helps ensure that you never have to wear your feelings again.

Reach for a life of joy and peace and growth and freedom. Reach for the life you really want.

Acceptance

It's called food addiction for a reason. It's physical. Your body is sensitive to refined, processed, and man-made foods. Much like the shape of your eyebrows or the strength of your vision, it's not something you chose. Accepting this truth is the hardest part.

When you accept something, you see it as it is.

Acceptance does not mean you surrender to the will of another. It doesn't mean you accept abuse or mistreatment and forego your boundaries, hopes, or dreams. In fact, when you accept what is, when you allow it to be and stop struggling against its existence, you learn how to take care of yourself and where to set boundaries.

> **When you accept what is, when you allow it to be and stop struggling against its existence, you learn how to take care of yourself and where to set boundaries.**

To give you an example, I hate going to the dentist. But when I have a toothache, I have two choices: deny it and let it get worse, or call the dentist and make an appointment. If I refuse to accept the fact that I have a toothache, the problem gets worse until I am forced to handle it. And that may mean a cap or a root canal, rather than just a filling. Refusal to accept and act costs me more time, more pain, and often more money.

When you are learning to accept your situation, a couple of emotions may arise that will do little more than swirl inside, torment, maybe even make you sick, and keep you from freedom: resistance and resentment. Let them in—then release them. Accepting your feelings is part of the package.

Resistance is a natural response; when you resist something, you are trying to protect yourself. In reality, you end up doing more harm than good. When you dig your heels in and refuse to acknowledge the root cause of the issue, refuse to take action, you waste time and energy and make things harder. You create anguish. So, while it may be unfair, unreasonable, someone else's fault, the result of other people's selfish actions, or plain bad luck, you have the power to change. The key to recovery is accepting where you are and finding what is needed to set yourself free.

Resentment is when you know something or someone has hurt you, and you're angry about it! Your "nemesis" may be inanimate; it may have power over the people or things you love, and you may not be strong enough to stop it. Worse yet, it may blame you for the problem, and you can't prove that it is not your fault. (If you have sexual abuse in your history, you can likely relate.)

Resentments have roots that grow deeper and deeper, wrapping around the spirit so you can't move freely and make good decisions. You may not even understand the whole problem or your role in it, but it can stay for years, to the point that it feels normal. That's why it's so important to face it, so you can free yourself and reclaim your joy.

Accept the things that you find true for you about food and eating, even though you do not like them or want them to be true. Set aside your resistance to the things you dislike and know that there is a better way.

Surrender

When you think of surrender, you may think of something like the surrender at Appomattox at the end of the Civil War. General Grant and General Lee first met on April 9, 1865, but part of the Confederate army took until the end of April, or longer, to surrender. (And some of that surrender affects us today.) It was a process of change, much like our own surrender. We want to make a change, yet we also want to enjoy a certain kind of food; we want what it does for us; we want to be able to eat like everybody else. Parts of our hearts and minds do not agree, and it may take a long time for us to be able to accept and surrender entirely.

Yet the surrender we're talking about here is not a sign of failure or defeat, as it is in times of war. It's a decision. It's a change of heart that leads to a commitment—and it's the key to creating the joyful, peaceful life you have always wanted, free of the obsession with food, eating, and body weight. Rather than waving a white flag, it's a call to positive action and a way to take back your power.

A better way of thinking about it may be found at the car lot. When you buy a new car, you surrender the title and ownership of your old clunker to the dealer, then you drive off with a shiny new convertible. When you let go of something that no longer works for you, you're able to get something even better.

Surrender is about reaching for something different—something you really want—and making the decision not to look back. Do you go back to the dealership to visit your old car? I doubt it, even if you miss its comfort and familiarity.

The logic is simple, but the practice is often difficult.

It may require some actionable steps. For example, you may need to find a place of quiet where you meditate on your surrender. Write down the problem: list all the issues; complain about how difficult it is. Write down the goal: what do you most want and need; what do you want to accomplish; what are the advantages, disadvantages, and consequences; what situations, solutions, and programs can help? Once you have it all down on paper, seek out others who have experienced the same problem or who are trained to help you solve it.

Sometimes it just helps to express concerns to a sympathetic ear—up to a point. If you give them a voice, give them a time limit. Prolonged or frequent venting can lend momentum to such feelings. Also, be aware of your audience. You want to seek out those who will listen, but ultimately help you to say, "Yes, yes, I accept that this is a terrible situation, and the way I can make it better is . . ."

Ultimately, surrender is calm and peaceful. It allows you to set down your anger, frustration, and failures to look for real answers to the problem. No doubt you'll experience other areas of growth as well. (Fixing the food problem often provides the opportunity to work on other problems, too; be sure to get effective help for all of them.)

Surrender is a process of your choosing, changing, and decision making. Surrender takes time. Give yourself a chance to plow through the hard parts and see how to get what you really want. Many of my clients have chosen a space of time (six months, a year, the fifth step, all twelve steps) to give themselves fully to this process before they decide whether they want to keep it.

Of course, we are imperfect beings, so total, ongoing, and permanent surrender is unrealistic. You may revert to your old way of thinking, particularly under stress, but it's important you remind yourself that surrender is not giving up on life but giving up on fighting with life. When you're not fighting it, you're working with it. And each day will bring a thousand little victories, all thanks to surrender.

EXERCISE: Surrender

It often helps to have a "Simple Surrender Statement" so you know what you are committing to. Here is an example. Change it any way you wish, then use it every day, every time you need it.

I have a major problem with _____ (food, eating, body weight, bingeing, self-hatred, etc.).

What I have tried before has not worked. Beginning today, for the next six months, I am going to work on this program in every way I can. Then I will re-evaluate and change if needed.

I want a life of _____ (peace, joy, freedom, etc.) from _____ (the food, obsessions, cravings, struggle, etc.).

I intend to focus my energies on the positive and stop fighting with my body and my mind and my life.

I intend to listen to the advice of others who have solved this problem and investigate what works for me.

I am not the most powerful being or force in the universe. I give permission to the forces in the universe to help me.

Rewrite this in your own words and change it any time you think you need to.

The Core of Your Recovery

Once you have accepted the problem and surrendered to change, you must make a serious decision to put your recovery at the center of your life choices and build the rest of your life around it. It's as pure and simple (and scary) as that.

Recovery requires more than following a special food plan. The purpose of the food plan is to move abusive foods far enough out of the way so you can begin to create the life you really want. It's a physical, mental, emotional, and spiritual change deeply tied to your identity.

That means your sense of self will be questioned. *Who is the real me; who am I determined to become?* That person is the one you must focus on from this point forward. That person is the one for whom you set aside your addictive foods and thoughts and behaviors; why you work to resolve deep-seated issues; why you seek outside help—from others, the universe, a Higher Power.

It requires work and practice to learn how to do this; it takes time to adjust and refocus.

And that is the goal of the Sane Food Solution: to get the insanity and craziness that have affected your life—through programs, exercises, and diets that do not work—out of your life; to find a new and comfortable and compassionate way of living and eating; to heal your body, mind, and spirit; and to create the life you have always wanted and dreamed of.

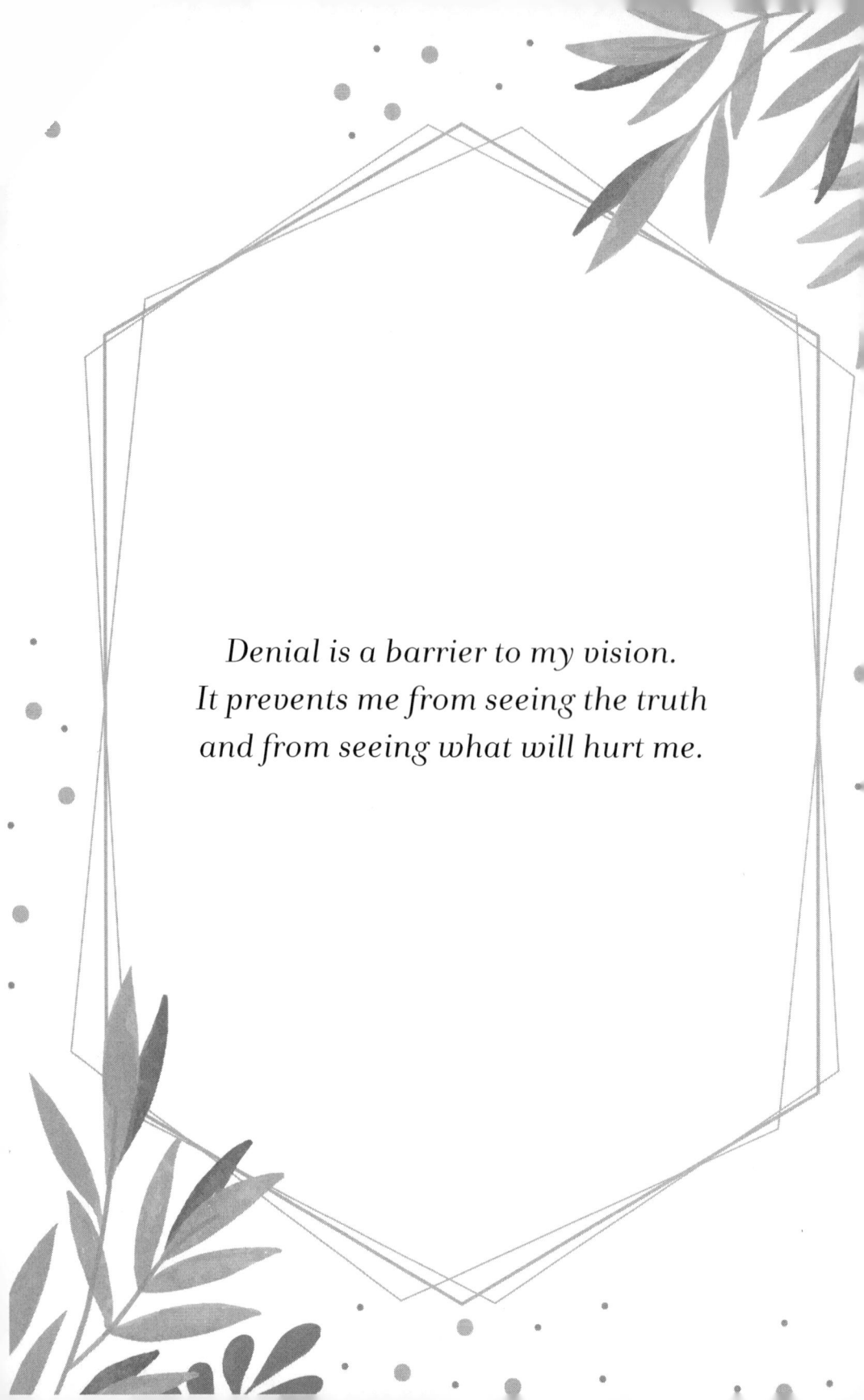

*Denial is a barrier to my vision.
It prevents me from seeing the truth
and from seeing what will hurt me.*

Chapter 3
Embracing Abstinence

Disclaimer: the food addiction problem looks different for everyone and may well change along with your life situation. That said, let's begin to look at the solution.

I want you to be very clear on this point: addiction is a force that functions in your mind and heart separately from your conscious thought or will. You may often feel like you have another voice in your mind, and sometimes it takes over your conscious thought. That's true. You do. Learning to handle this other force is essential to your recovery. To recover, you need to take control of what you eat and what you don't. I call this "food abstinence," but it's not about starvation or crash diets. It's about learning how your body responds to certain foods and abstaining from what does you harm, replacing them with life-supporting options. This is the essence of the Sane Food Plan.

Oh, good, you may think, *I can do abstinence. I'm an old pro at strict diets.*

The Pendulum Swing

There's a pattern: first you starve—you diet, restrict foods, count calories, eat the pre-packaged food from a weight-loss program, purge, overexercise, or take diuretics or diet pills; then, you stuff—you binge, eat double portions, stop for two muffins and a breakfast sandwich, down a half gallon of ice cream in front of the TV, whatever.

Diets and binges, and the swing between both, stir control issues. When you binge, you may feel out of control. When you diet, you may feel controlled. Diets are, by nature, restrictive. You eat what someone else tells you to eat, when they tell you to eat it, and you don't enjoy it. When you diet, it must be perfect. It must be exactly right, lined up neatly on a plate. When you binge, you can eat anything you want in copious amounts. You can wolf down that food, not noticing, not listening. Who cares if the donuts are days old?

When you diet, there is never enough food, but when you binge, there is still never enough food. When you diet, you feel deprived, but when you binge? You may not think you're feeling deprived, but I suggest you do. You feel deprived of love and hope and other good feelings. Do you see how it's all mixed up?

Back and forth you go, all the while feeling tense, anxious, defensive, irritable, and hopeless, praying you won't gain another thirty pounds during the next round. When you binge, it feels ugly. When you diet, it feels shameful. Binges are about self-hatred; dieting is about self-hatred. The next binge, and it always comes, is not necessarily a quick fix for your weight, but it's probably a quick fix for your feelings. When you binge, you do so to feel excited and alive; when you diet, you do so to feel alive, as well. On and on it goes.

In other words, dieting and bingeing are opposite sides of the same coin, and they take you to the same place: defeat, despair, and failure.

Abstinence: The Middle Way

Abstinence is the place in the middle. It's where you're not starving or bingeing but circumventing cravings and obsessions because you are learning to live free of addictive substances while meeting your body's nutrient needs.

It allows for enough space to live and enjoy your life. Your boundaries shouldn't be too tight, which will drive you back to bingeing out of hunger, or too loose, which will start the cycle again because you haven't thoroughly eliminated your trigger foods.

Gaining control of your eating and recovering from food addiction requires a serious physical process of growth and change. It takes time and energy to learn to eat abstinently. There will be ups and downs, adjustments that need to be made. Controlling your choices and managing what you say to yourself is vital. Be gentle with yourself. A change in behavior also requires a change in attitude toward yourself. It means treating the body with respect and meeting its needs for food, rest, exercise, and other supports.

Your Commitment

What you think in your mind comes true in your life. That's why abstinence begins with a simple statement of intent:

"Beginning today..." Not tomorrow, not next week, not on Monday, like every other diet program. Now. Enough: here is where it ends and where I start. I've gone down this path often enough. I am done.

> **Beginning today, I commit myself to learning how to live a joyful, useful life without abusing my body, mind, or spirit with food, or thoughts, or other drugs.**

"I commit myself..." A commitment is a pledge; it binds you to a certain course. In this case, it's a course of your choosing. You, yourself, are committing to who you are and what you want. It's not some external straitjacket someone tied to you. It's not the rule of another. Abstinence bubbles up from inside you, asking you to make different, better choices with the goal of creating your core recovery—of walking on sacred ground; of creating a life beyond your wildest dreams, the life you really want.

Remember, you make the decisions here. You're not a wayward child. (I cringe when I hear clients say, "I am not allowed..." or "I allowed myself...") You're making the decision to move your food life onto a different path, with different goals and priorities. This is your commitment to yourself. All your life, others have given you their dieting solutions. In abstinence, you are committing yourself to find or create the solutions that are right for you.

"To learning..." Since abstinence and recovery are a journey, not a destination, this is the most important piece. You will need to make many choices, changes, and detours along the way. It will open you up to a series of growth experiences. So, commit yourself to the process of learning how to live life differently. At least agree to work on it, knowing you won't be perfect at it, and the path will be created as you go. Some blunders and absurdities will creep in, no doubt. Your addiction will fight you every step of the way. Your friends, family, and colleagues will not understand and may not know how to be effectively supportive. You may be unsure what to do next. That is okay.

"To live a joyful, useful life..." This is, in my opinion, the best reason to attempt abstinence. The life you get with abstinence is so much better than the life you will have without it. It's worth the sacrifice. It frees you from the obsession with food, eating, dieting, and body weight that has distracted you from creating the life you want, need, and deserve. Think about what food has taken from you, even though that can be painful or scary. Think how different your life might have been if it were not for the food issues. Think how different your life could be if they were out of the way. Food may have been a tool that allowed you to survive in the past, but now it's keeping you from what you really want. The primary purpose of abstinence is to change that—to turn despair to joy.

"Without abusing . . ." This is where the rubber meets the road. This is absolutely critical to abstinence. It matters not the addiction—food, gambling, sex, compulsive shopping, shoplifting, alcohol, Xanax, mental obsessions, computer games—it will use anything to maintain a foothold in your life. You need to confront the real issues.

You must stop hurting yourself. No more self-abuse. Not with food, not with thoughts, not with other drugs or obsessions. You must stop using food to hurt your body, mind, and spirit. You may not be able to do it at first. You may need to learn this skill. Restrictive diets are just as abusive as binges and purges. They hurt you. They demean you. And they distract you from your real goal.

No more self-abuse.

The Building Blocks of Abstinence

Start with Your Core of Recovery. This is your decision, your surrender, to learn to do the things that will allow you to maintain your abstinence:

1. Nutrient-rich food that meets the body's needs
2. Enough food so you are satisfied at the end of each meal or snack

3. Freedom from the foods that compromise your abstinence and your goals
4. Freedom from abusive food behaviors
5. Skills to manage life and feelings without food
6. Space for emotional and spiritual growth

Now, let's take a closer look at each of these characteristics . . .

1. To recover from years of self-abuse with food, you must give your body all the nutrients it needs at the time of day it needs them most. This means high-quality, nutrient-rich foods with lots of calcium and B vitamins and reasonable amounts of healthy fats and everything else your body best uses to repair, replace, and restore itself. You need these nutritious foods in the right amounts. The way you eat has a major effect on the structure and function of your body, and we need to repair the damage that has been created by abusive eating. You may need supplements in the beginning, but eventually you will rely solely on whole foods, real foods, under-processed foods, and high-nutrient foods—as close as you can get them to the way God and Mother Nature planned them.

2. Most of the time, diets do not give you enough nutrients to allow the body to maintain its structure and function adequately. That is one of the reasons you keep struggling against yourself. If you're hungry, you will struggle; if you have too few nutrients or the food plan is not balanced for you, you will have a hard time overriding the body's urges. Physiology is stronger than willpower, 99.999% of the time. You want to have enough food so that you are not

hungry most of the time. You want to feel hungry ten to fifteen minutes before a meal, and after the meal, be able to say, "Ah, that was good. That was enough."

3. What are the foods that make your abstinence and your life harder? Which foods make you feel better one minute and worse the next? Which foods sabotage your recovery efforts? We call these your drug and trigger foods. They vary, but one symptom is the same all the time: when you start eating a drug food, you're unable to stop. Drug foods are going to be different foods for different people, and everyone is going to have a different threshold for the kinds and amounts of foods they can eat and tolerate. But whatever food sets you off, you need to deal with it.

4. Freedom from abusive food behaviors means no bingeing, purging, or starving; no double portions, or restrictive portions. More than that, it means a change in your attitude toward yourself. It means treating the body with gentleness and respect and meeting its needs for food, rest, exercise, and other supports.

Most people understand abstinence from foods that trigger binges, but they don't understand how abstinence from behaviors fits in. Certain food behaviors can be problems for you, too—for example, eating standing up, eating while preparing food, or skipping meals. This means no getting out of bed in the middle of the night to eat in private; no obsessive calculating; fitting in the Key Lime Pie; "allowing" yourself to have a piece of that drug food; punishing yourself with laxatives, overexercise, or overwork. It means you will no longer be a compliant victim and then punish yourself for it.

5. Without using food to manage feelings or to hurt or punish yourself, how do you fill that dark, empty place where food used to be; how do you participate in work functions, friendships, and relationships; how do you handle sorrow, joy, and holidays? You need to begin a process of treating the body, mind, and spirit with respect. In doing so, you will learn new ways to manage old problems and set yourself free from them.

6. Recovery means you change to become the person you want to be. An important aspect of this is to leave room for emotional and spiritual growth. Connecting to a Higher Power of your choice allows you to get in touch with the ageless, timeless, eternal you. Or, if you'd prefer a more down to earth reason, it provides long-standing spiritual principles to help you heal, forgive, and connect with others; it offers a sense of serenity and a different perspective on life's obstacles.

This is abstinence and recovery. This is how you can break free. When you draw such abstinence boundaries, you come up with a plan that is very different from any diet you have ever used for weight loss or weight gain.

Abstinence is a Process

The solution to your eating problem is yours alone; it's unique to you. If you look only at the symptom, your weight or body shape, you may find a temporary solution in a diet or weight loss plan. If you want to solve your unique eating problem, however, you need to identify problematic food.

Now, an all or nothing approach is often very difficult or creates additional problems. So, let your recovery be done in stages, gently, beginning with showing respect for the needs of your body, as well as those of your spirit. Taste, enjoy, and savor healthy food; enter the process of growing strong enough to taste, enjoy, and savor your recovery life.

The first step in this process is to take an inventory of sorts: what trigger foods are in your home? Remove them if you can; if others eat them, adjust cabinets and cupboards to keep them out of your line of sight.

Next, make an initial plan: decide what foods you will eat; maybe make a trip to the grocery store. Talk to the people you live with and tell them what you are planning—they may want to try it with you. Ask for the behavior changes and cooperation you will need. And know what you'll do, who you will call, if you need additional support.

Then, when you're ready, begin. You can start small by drinking adequate fluids (unsweetened and without artificial sweeteners). Most people need about eight cups of fluid per day.

From there, you can choose a food plan and begin to follow it: one food at a time, one meal at a time, one hour at a time. For example, you may want to try *Your Personal Food Plan Guide: The Sane Food Solution.* You'll find information on this at the back of the book. You may also choose to see a dietitian, a nutritionist, or another advocate you trust, or find a book, physician, sponsor, or program to guide you.

And take note of what happens. If you're not feeling safe, or not seeing the results you're after, make changes as needed. If your binge foods are pushing their way in, kick them to the curb. Check out the "Withdrawal Symptoms" in the appendix. Are you feeling withdrawal; what do you need to keep going in this abstinence program; what do you need now?

Reach out for the help and support you need. And be gentle with yourself.

> **EXERCISE: Your recovery baseline**

Before you start the work required to address your food addiction, you'll want to know your baseline, or your starting point. It helps you know what needs to be done—and see your progress along the way.

1. List five foods that trouble you, that you eat too much, crave a lot, feel like you can't stop eating.
2. What time of day is it usually when you crave them?
3. What kind of textures do you prefer?
4. What makes you stop eating these foods?
5. What feelings usually come up when you binge or eat badly?
6. What are you saying to yourself at this time?

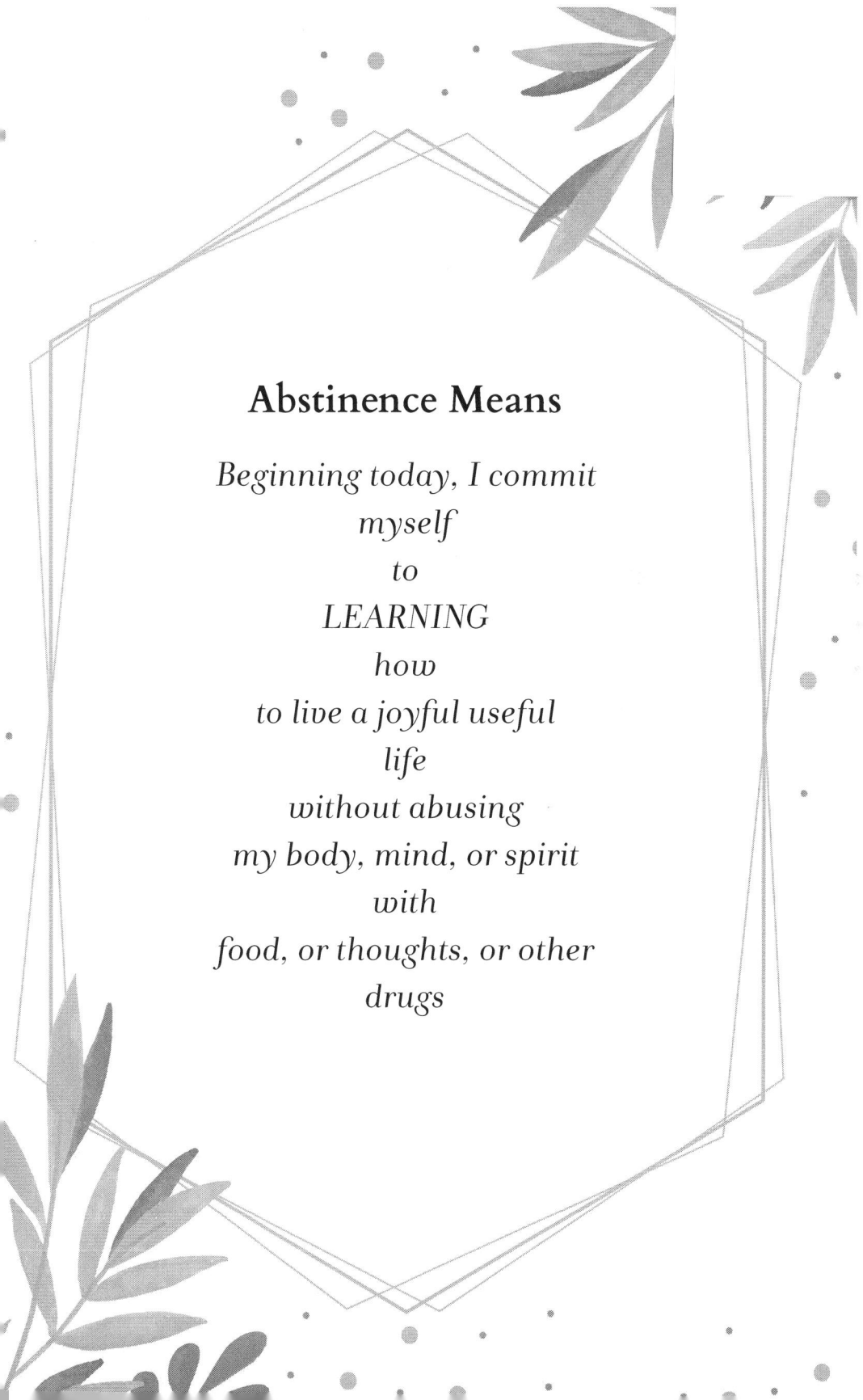

Abstinence Means

Beginning today, I commit
myself
to
LEARNING
how
to live a joyful useful
life
without abusing
my body, mind, or spirit
with
food, or thoughts, or other
drugs

Chapter 4

Freedom from Trigger, Drug, and Binge Foods

Abstinence requires that you get addictive foods far enough out of the way that you can create the life that you want and replace the addictive foods with foods that support your physical, emotional, and spiritual well-being; abstinence also instills food behaviors that unhook you from abusive habits and rituals that drive a wedge between you and true connection. That's the whole point of creating a strong and rewarding recovery program, the point of the recovery process.

But you don't want to immediately pull these foods out of your diet; right now, you simply want to identify them. Without preparing the body and mind beforehand, eliminating these substances will only trigger a physical reaction, and cravings will refuse to go away. Just like that, you'll be right back on the pendulum, swinging—especially if you experience a stressor or a situation that triggers

> **Without preparing the body and mind beforehand, eliminating these substances will only trigger a physical reaction, and cravings will refuse to go away.**

addictive eating behaviors. So, it's important you recognize the three types of problematic foods.

Drug Foods: Drugs tend to serve a purpose—they manage many diseases; they may help us heal and feel better; they may protect us or support the body in its work. They are often used for healing, pain relief, and helping the body maintain its health and well-being. Drug foods, in our context, are very different. They dull painful or unwelcome emotions. They help us avoid dealing with frightening situations or powerful feelings.

In the beginning, they may have provided some comfort, support, or healing. They may well have been a part of your family's life, customs, or ritual. Now, their reactions in your brain have changed, and they are different. They are not healing or helpful. They may provide temporary relief, but that comes with a price—their consequences. You know a food is a drug for you when it calls to you, when it takes up residence in your mind, makes demands, and makes you uncomfortable. Drug foods glow for you. When you start eating them, you find yourself unable to stop. There is never enough. They are never rich enough, salty enough, or sweet enough. A drug food is eaten in relatively large amounts to medicate an urgency to eat signaled from the brain. Drug foods are going to be different for everyone because they're based on personal preferences and experiences. They might be smooth, creamy, chocolatey, crispy, crunchy, or salty like potato chips. They might be creamy and crunchy, like ice cream with nuts in it or chips with lots of guacamole and sour cream. Drug foods can be known—you may go for ice cream after an emotional upheaval—but they can also be hidden from view. Processed foods often contain addictive ingredients that spur overeating. Manufacturers depend on this to keep you buying more. Usually, the nutrient content is limited, and the inclusion of extra sugar, salt, and chemical additives may increase your appetite and tolerance.

Trigger Foods: These foods set off the need to eat abusively. Certain calorie-dense foods, especially those loaded with refined sugars, can trigger overeating and cause you to overindulge. Again, food manufacturers include ingredients that trigger overeating, but the smell (or the sight) of a particular food can compel you to overeat as well. If you anchored the smell of pancakes to childhood sexual abuse, for instance, you may find yourself eating anything you can get your hands on just to quell the feelings of rage and hopelessness.

Binge Foods: These foods are eaten in large amounts—a gallon of ice cream, an entire pizza, a bag of potato chips, or a big bowl of popcorn. You know for a fact that these foods work for you when you need comfort, when you want nothing more than to tamp down unwanted feelings. These are your go-to foods.

Here's an example of how these three problematic food types work together.

One of my clients went out to dinner with friends, and they brought a bottle of their special wine. "You have to try this," they said. So, like a polite friend, she had a small glass. When it came time for dessert, my client was used to ordering a cup of coffee or tea. That night, she could not resist the chocolate cheesecake. It was as though the wine had opened the floodgates to her resistance. After her husband went to bed that evening, she felt compelled to have a huge serving of ice cream, and not just any ice cream—Very Chocolate ice cream—because the cheesecake wasn't chocolatey enough. In this scenario, the wine was the trigger, the cheesecake was the drug (at least, it was supposed to be the substance that quieted her brain), and the ice cream was the binge.

Food Categories Common to Addiction

Anything you insert into your oral cavity can lead to addiction, but some work harder than others. Here are ten of the most frequent culprits:

- Sugar, in all its forms
- Fats
- Flours
- Salt
- Caffeine
- Alcohol
- Chocolate
- Artificial Sweeteners
- Volume
- Texture

Let's talk about each a bit to give you a better understanding . . .

Sugar, as glucose in the body, is a simple carbohydrate. It's a natural product to the body, used to maintain functionality. The brain only runs on sugar, so the body can make glucose from every food you eat, from butter to prime rib.

That's what makes high-sugar foods one of the biggest problems and the hardest to deal with. Realistically, it's not possible to eat an entirely sugar-free food plan. But if you're a "sugar addict"—meaning, sugar is the primary ingredient that sets off abusive eating—cutting back is a good place to start.

Rather than avoid the offending product altogether (as would be suggested if you were addicted to heroin), you want to create ways to present appropriate carbohydrates to the body in the proper amounts so the body can handle it effectively.

You have your own threshold; if you go over that amount, your body will get triggered. So, if you are sensitive to sugar, the trick is to get your sugar intake low enough, to get your carbohydrate intake low enough, to ensure you won't be triggered. And if you provide the carbohydrates evenly throughout the day, or in the way that works best for your body, you should not feel "peaks and valleys" in your energy level.

Also, be aware. Fruits naturally contain the sugars fructose and glucose in different amounts, but when the fructose is separated from the glucose in digestion, it can be stored as fat in the liver (and can even create or contribute to fatty liver disease). This doesn't happen when you simply eat fruit. However, problems arise when the fructose is highly concentrated, as in high-fructose corn syrup (HFCS).

High-fructose corn syrup is cheap, shelf stable, and can be used to improve the texture of baked goods. Dr. George Bray and Dr. Nicole Aveena have carefully studied its effects on the body. In rats, those given HFCS gained significantly more weight than those who were given glucose. In the famous "Dr Pepper study," those who drank soda sweetened with HFCS had twenty percent more fructose in their blood than those who didn't. This is likely because when fruit concentrates are created, the fiber and many of the vitamins are taken away, leaving behind only the sugar.[1]

There is a catch. Your tolerance level can change with stress and other activities. For instance, I have a client who is violently sensitive

---

[1]. Nicole M. Avena, *Sugarless: A 7-Step Plan to Uncover Hidden Sugars, Curb Your Cravings, and Conquer Your Addiction* (Union Square & Co, 2023), 54 and 57.

to sugar. Small amounts of sugar in her foods can really trigger her. Yet she ran the Hawaii Marathon, which involved hours of physical activity. She used sugar-containing gels, and they did not bother her during the marathon; her body burned those calories in the physical activity; there was nothing left. We calculated very carefully the amount of carbohydrates she needed per hour so her body would use that carbohydrate effectively. She will not touch them in her daily life.

You must learn to listen to the body and adjust to what the body is telling you. If you are under a lot of stress, you may find that your threshold is lower. You may need to be more careful—not more indulgent—when you are under stress.

There are more than 160 names for sugar on my list (see this at www.sanefood.com/bonus/), and I am certain that more names will be created and revealed by the manufacturers.

Fat is an essential nutrient for the body. It's an essential part of many cells. It's an essential part of your brain structure (sixty-seven percent of the weight of your brain is likely to be fat-based). Your nerves are covered with a layer of protein and fat. Your skin is constructed of three layers of protein and one layer of fat. Your hair is fat entwined around protein. Take all the fat out of your diet, and your skin will dry out; your hair will get dry, brittle, and fall out; your nails will become soft and peel and break; you will have no energy; and your libido will move south for the duration. If it continues, you may find it difficult to think clearly. And if you have been on many fat-free diets, these symptoms may make it harder to get better.

In the 1970s, fat was the food to remove from a food plan. No Longer. We have seen that this does not work long-term. Now we know the body needs a particular amount of fat each day. For example, polyunsaturated and monounsaturated vegetable oils are the raw materials with which the body makes estrogen, progesterone, testosterone, and thyroxin, which are the major marker regulatory hormones in the body. They are the hormones that run your body, so you need to present the right fats in the right amounts. When you set up your food plan to give you enough of the right kind, you change or eliminate the ones that cause you trouble.

Flour consists of 150 to 1,000 molecules of sugar hooked together. I have not met anyone who is sensitive to sugar who is not also sensitive to white or whole wheat flour at some level. White flour has had the bran (the tough outer hull) and the germ (the part that will grow the new plant) removed. That means all the fiber, protein, B vitamins, and minerals have been removed. Only the starch, the strings of sugar molecules, remains.

Enriched wheat flour has three B vitamins and one mineral added—only because people got deficiency diseases when flour began to be refined this way. The other fourteen B vitamins, three minerals, protein, and fiber, which are in the whole grain kernel, are lost.

There is also a portion issue here. The average restaurant-size portion of pasta is about three cups. What other foods do people regularly choose to eat in a six-serving size portion? (Six four-ounce potatoes, perhaps, or six small ears of corn?)

You could be sensitive to flour, or to wheat, or to gluten, or to all three. We will work on these issues in a later chapter, but for now, if you have some unspecified sensitivity, you will eventually want to take out all flour from all sources—white flour, whole wheat flour, rye flour, spinach flour, tapioca starch, and corn meal.

Salt is a sneaky substance. The body needs salt to function. Yet increase your salt intake, and your body holds more water; your blood pressure goes up; the hormone adrenalin is released by the adrenals, which causes the release of insulin; insulin lowers blood sugar, which makes you feel hungry; and your feeling of hunger triggers a binge.

It is recommended that we consume about 2,000 milligrams of sodium per day; our average intake is estimated to be between 6,000 and 12,000 milligrams of sodium per day. If you're sensitive to salt, you may be consuming even more. So, while some sodium is essential to the body, you need a plan to keep it in safe amounts.

Caffeine may be a substance you need to watch, too. What kind of caffeine could be problematic? "The kind that comes in my coffee cup every morning, with a good dose of sugar and half-and-half!" says my client. "It's an antioxidant, like a pomegranate in disguise," she adds. All joking aside, the evidence is pretty clear: two to four eight-ounce cups of regular coffee a day has no negative effect. It's when you find yourself drinking eighteen cups of regular coffee a day that issues arise: your veins contract, which raises blood pressure; your adrenals release insulin, which lowers glucose, which makes you hungry. Caffeine in large amounts may make you more anxious and irritable and keep you from adequate sleep and rest. And remember, coffee cannot count as your fluid allowance. The creamers and sweeteners used often have lots of calories—and, no, it's not an antioxidant!

Alcohol is the ultimate sugar. Take sugar and ferment it (or let it rot), and you've got alcohol. Alcohol and sugar alcohols are powerful triggers for people sensitive to sugar. Some can handle a glass of wine with dinner; most cannot. Even foods cooked in an alcohol-based sauce can trigger a sugar addict since only about forty percent of the alcohol burns off during cooking.

Alcohol is high in calories and nutrient-free, but what causes problems for a compulsive eater is that it tends to reduce inhibitions and cloud judgments. This makes it so much easier to make poor decisions about food and the other issues in your life. Clients often call alcohol a "gateway food." More than once I've heard, "It's what I consume before I really get in trouble."

Chocolate can be a very effective drug food, but most often in combination with other drug or trigger foods. Chocolate is special for several reasons. Milk chocolate has tryptophan in it, which helps release serotonin. Chocolate has fat in it, which helps release endorphins, which are the pain relievers in your brain; it also contains caffeine, which releases adrenalin and enhances the addictive system; and it usually comes with sugar, which is likely to be another addictive drug for you.

Chocolate has one additional property. It releases dopamine, which is your extra special feel wonderful hormone. Other things that effectively release dopamine are cocaine and nicotine. Cocaine and nicotine may be more harmful to the body in other ways, but sensitivity to chocolate can be as strong and pervasive—and as difficult to resolve.

Artificial Sweeteners are so addictive, but what makes them so? Is it the sweet taste, the combination with other products? A number of my clients use sweeteners to excess—two to three liters of diet soda a day, seventy to eighty of those little packets. Those little packets also may contain maltodextrin and dextrose, which are each a kind of sugar. Often people can handle small amounts without difficulty, but a large quantity equals a large dose of both the sweetener and the sugar analogs. And that can be a problem.

Using four to six packets and drinking one or two diet sodas a day might be a reasonable amount for you, depending on your priorities and situation. However, they may cause the same effect on your brain neurotransmitters as the real sugar products; they may provide the same jolt. Honor your own individual uniqueness in this and deal with the issue in the way that works best for you.

For a safety report on your favorite sweetener, go to the bonus material at www.sanefood.com/bonus.

Volume may be an issue if you live in fear of being hungry. For some food abusers, it doesn't really matter what the food is; they just want more . . . and more . . . and more! Do you feel the need to finish the entire box or bag; do you buy smaller sizes thinking you will eat less—when you buy Halloween candy, do you need to buy it a second time? When you look at your weighed and measured food, do you pray it will be enough; when you start a new food plan and take out certain foods, do you resist weighing and measuring because you're afraid you'll starve? Do you eat unrestricted amounts of the foods labeled acceptable? Do you wake in the middle of the night, stuffed and sick, with a horrible "volume burp" that feels like the food is coming back up? Is it easy for you to "diet" in the mornings because you're still full from the previous nights' binge?

If you answered yes to any of these questions, volume (or, more importantly, a fear of being hungry) may be a problem, and you may need to weigh and measure some or all your foods. This sounds painful, but it's really a magical tool that gives you power over your food intake and recovery process. It makes your proportions of different food match the body's needs. After years of struggle with food and body weight, lots of people can lose the ability to tell how much is enough. Now you can feel satisfied at the end of the meal. The right proportions adjust your satisfaction and fit your body. So, weigh and measure till your eyeballs get adjusted to choosing the right amounts.

Textures can be the downfall of some food addicts. Maybe it's smooth and creamy: ice cream, peanut butter, pudding—something cool and soothing going down. From the moment you put it in your mouth, you can feel yourself relax and calm down. Maybe it's crunchy and salty. You lie to yourself by hiding crumbled tortilla chips in the middle of your healthy green salad.

Vegetables will do in a pinch, but not as well. You buy the baked chips, and act as though they are healthier (they're not fried), then hide the real stuff from the family. After a long, hard day, you release the tension with chips, pretzels, crackers, or popcorn . . . as long as you are alone. Or maybe it's creamy and crunchy together? It may be almost a ritual: first the sweet and creamy, then the salty and crunchy, then the sweet and creamy again. When you're so stuffed you cannot see straight, you realize you did it again.

> ## EXERCISE: Identify your binge, drug, and trigger foods

It is important for you to know what foods and what ingredients set off your struggle with foods. Individual triggers can be combined to create even more possibilities. What are your drug, trigger, and binge foods? They vary for everybody, but the symptoms associated with their consumption don't. For right now, simply notice which foods set you off; look for commonalities—and be honest.

In a peaceful place, with no one asking you for your attention, take a close look at the foods you're eating: what they're made of, their characteristics, what they have in common. To get started, write down your answers to the following questions:

- Which high-calorie, nutrient-free foods do you crave?

    Make a list of them and include all their friends. (If Doritos trigger you, Tostitos and other chips will too!)

- What are these foods made of (sugar, flour, salt, fat; creamy, crunchy, a mixture of both)?

- What are the foods you cannot stop eating?

- Write yourself a list of ten or fifteen (if you only have a few, that's okay).

- What foods call to you when you are at the convenience store, upset, or up late at night?

- What foods are similar?

    Be specific: potato chips or tortilla chips; chocolate chip cookies or Double Stuf Oreos; clams or crabs; Aunt Sarah's or Sara Lee; bologna, salami, liverwurst, or sausage; pasta with marinara or with Alfredo sauce; things that come in plastic that are four bites and four hundred calories. Butterfingers or Milky Ways or Snickers?

- What foods really do it for you; what really sets you off?

- What about texture—what texture does it for you (smooth and creamy, crunchy, maybe a combination)?

- What food categories are most likely to contain your drug or trigger foods?

Once you've written down your list of trigger foods, scrutinize a bit further because your triggers may not be quite what you think. To get at the real culprit, you need to be honest and specific about wh egories of food set off your sensitivities. This can be tricky.

For example, let's say you listed bread and pasta as your primary trigger foods. Here's how you might get to the heart of the matter.

First, take a closer look at the bread: is it fresh baked or Italian crunchy bread, with butter or without? Is it the bread you desire, or is bread simply the vehicle with which you carry butter to your mouth? Is it white bread, with butter or brie?

Next, consider the pasta: can you eat a whole pound of pasta, even if you're full? Can you keep eating till it's gone? What is your preferred topping: salt; pepper; butter; olive oil; parmesan/Romano cheese—wine? Will you add shrimp or chicken, or leave it plain?

Your answers might indicate that your triggers are flour and fat, maybe salt. And from that, you can bet potato chips (also flour, fat, and salt) are triggers, too.

But what if peanut M&Ms are the first thing you reach for when stressed—is that sugar? For that, you need to look at your second and third favorite foods for emotional eating. In the interest of this example, let's say they're chocolate chip cookies and potato chips, respectively.

So, what do peanut M&M's and chocolate chip cookies have in common? Sugar and fat and chocolate. Would fat free hot cocoa work to satisfy the craving? Probably not. Would you rather have a Milky Way or a Snickers bar? Will a sugar-free Fudgsicle work for you, or does it have to be a real Fudgsicle with fat? Will you be able to eat only one, or will you want to eat the whole box?

The key is to satisfy your nutrient needs and calorie goals without triggering abusive eating—not blindly eliminating food categories that may not actually be the culprit.

As you look at your primary trigger foods, you are going to be able to see that, perhaps for you, it is sugar, fat, and chocolate. For someone else, it may be sugar and chocolate only. For another, the crunchy, nutty texture has real importance. Remember, addiction is also a physical sensitivity. When you want to escape from your reality or a negative situation, what foods do you fantasize indulging in?

> **Get to know which products are the most effective triggers for you.**

Get to know which products are the most effective triggers for you. If it's sugar, get to know the names for sugar, all one hundred and sixty of them. There are lots of foods that have sugar in them. The eventual goal is to reduce your intake of your personal trigger foods to the point where you are comfortable (that is, without cravings and tortured thoughts).

If you are sensitive to sugar, you'll want to take out any sugar that is not essential. Do you really need sugar in your salad dressing, butter, cottage cheese? What you need is to be free of cravings. So, eliminate the things that don't have a huge effect on you by themselves. For example, I do not need sugar as the first ingredient in my ketchup label. Buying ketchup that has sugar fifth or sixth on the ingredient list lowers my total sugar intake and gives me a bit more space without cravings; and it gets me more tomato-ey ketchup!

Typical Trigger Situations

Food triggers are not the only thing to be aware of; you also want to be aware of situations that can trigger binges.

A trigger situation can be internal or external. Internal situations include eating to manage painful situations or to silence negative feelings—anger, boredom, loneliness, fear, or sorrow. External situations may include dinner with your grandmother, which brings back memories of childhood abuse; the sound of that man's voice on the phone, which makes your heart thump and your stomach turn over; or your boss saying it's time for your annual review, and you just know.

Society is full of sensory triggers, too. You need only watch television to see a large amount of delicious food: those eating it right before your eyes are the perfect weight, gorgeous, and tastefully dressed; their children are all smiles—they never make a fuss or have tantrums. It's obvious you should go there and, "Make it Supersize!"

Speaking of advertising tactics, did you know that each time Cinnabon bakes cinnamon buns, they put a flavor packet in the oven? That packet is what fills the mall with the scent of baking cinnamon buns. If that scent causes you to head straight to a kiosk . . .

Be aware. Get to know the trigger situations you are going to have to live with and what that means for you.

> **Get to know the trigger situations you are going to have to live with and what that means for you.**

Once you recognize your trigger, drug, and binge foods, sit back and assess; what are the foods and ingredients you eventually need to remove from your food plan? Make your list. In a subsequent stage, you will take out all the foods you have trouble with and then take out all the foods that are like them. For example, if chips are a problem for you, all chips are likely to trigger you. If it looks like a chip and crunches like a chip, it is likely to trigger you.

For now, keep an eye out for them. Start reading food labels (we'll go into more depth on this subject in Chapter 9). Choose products with sugar listed low on the ingredient list and little or none of your "sensitive" foods wherever you easily can. Over time, this will make your life calmer and more peaceful. If you don't understand the label, or if it has ingredients that may hurt you or those you choose to avoid, don't buy it. It's a simple boundary. Put it back. Walk away. Say a prayer and set it out of your mind.

> **EXERCISE: List the trigger situations that trouble you most**

We will dedicate a whole chapter on trigger situations (including a toolbox for handling them); for now, make a list of your trigger situations so you are at least aware of them.

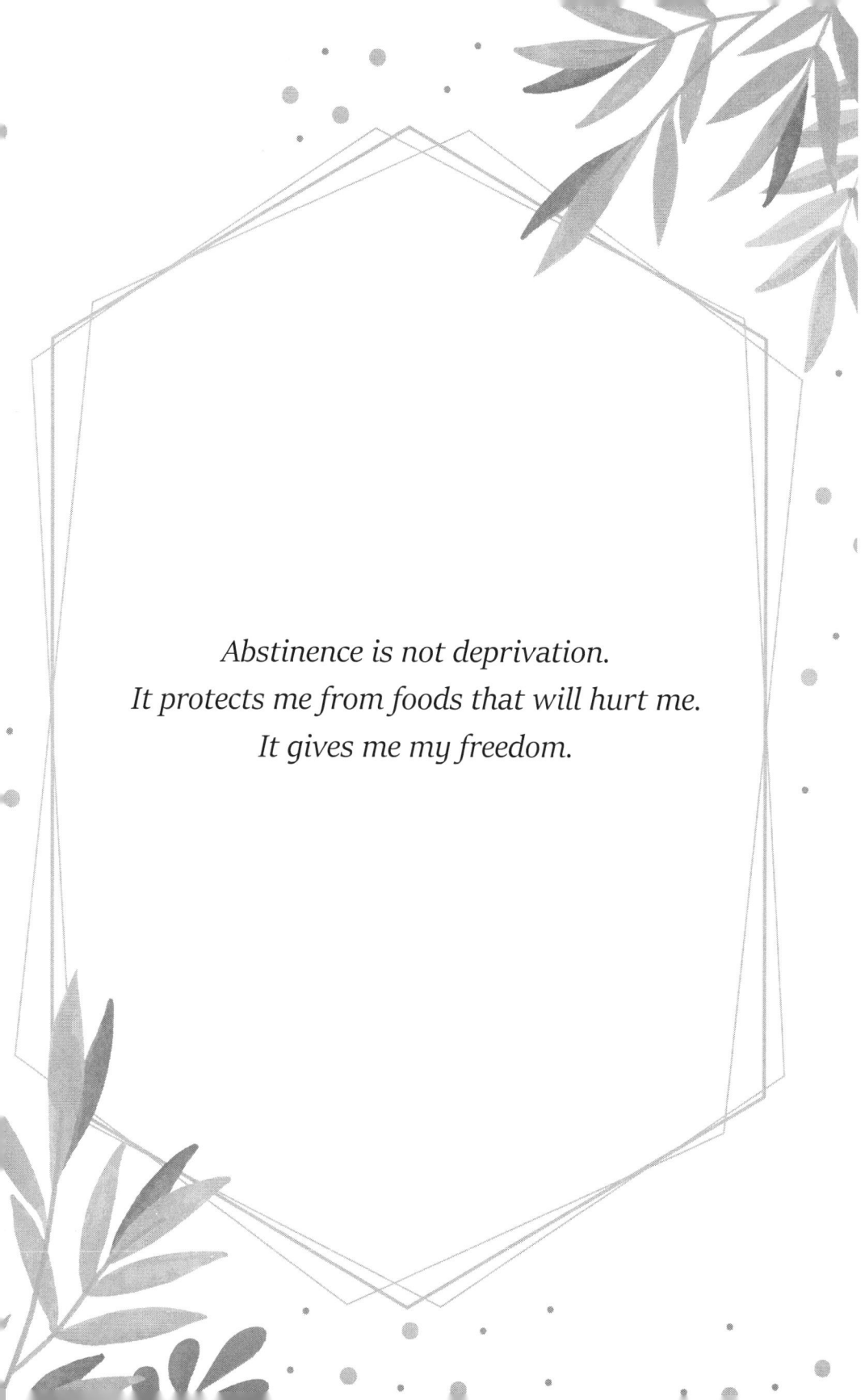

*Abstinence is not deprivation.
It protects me from foods that will hurt me.
It gives me my freedom.*

Chapter 5

Paving the Way

Most people, be they food addicts or not, are so used to diets they immediately look for the "six ounces of fruit, two ounces of protein, one ounce of cereal" instructions before they begin. The problem with those diets is that they're so rigid and so structured you can't stay on them for longer than six weeks (maybe even six days).

On the flip side, when you've been eating anything and everything, when you're desperate and desolate and you don't know what to do, and you feel like following a food plan is way too much work, let me put your mind at ease. The next thing we're going to do is create the outer limits of your food plan. We're going to interrupt your previous eating pattern by introducing key foods at certain times of day, even if you continue to eat problematic foods.

In the last chapter, we identified your binge, trigger, and drug foods, as well as your primary trigger situations. Taking this step by step, we'll now determine what to eat and drink and when to better prepare your body for the changes ahead.

Remember, a food plan without a structured recovery program will become another failed diet. The food plan needs to become a comfortable vehicle to take you where you want to go. I'll say this again and again, just so you don't forget.

You'll want to follow these simple guidelines impeccably, meticulously, determinedly, no matter what else you do. Understand me here: no matter what you eat or do not eat—whether you binge, purge, starve, over-exercise, eat all your "downfall" foods—whatever else you do, go to the next five behaviors immediately. (That means in the next five minutes, not on Monday.)

1. **Drink eight to ten cups of liquid every day**. Water, herbal tea, seltzer or soda water (including that flavored by lemon, lime, or mandarin orange), or other calorie-free, decaffeinated beverage is a good option. Any beverage artificially sweetened by the manufacturer, coffee, or diet soda does not count.

This is important. You've got to drink your fluids. If your body is losing weight, it will release ketone bodies, which go to your kidneys. Ketone bodies have ammonia in them. If you're not drinking enough water to wash those ketone bodies out of your kidneys, they'll move over to the liver, which will convert them to fat cells. And there goes your weight loss.

And the water you drink must be sugar-free. When you drink those sweet diet sodas, the body tastes the sweetness, and the brain thinks it's sugar. In response, it releases insulin to store fat. But since there are no calories, you wind up hungrier because the body has taken all the calories it can find out of your bloodstream and used them for something else. Once again, you don't lose weight.

Nearly every chemical reaction in your body requires some fluid, and dehydration can literally kill people. Please do not deprive your body of this essential substance!

Now, you may be wondering how much liquid you should be drinking. Some suggest you take your weight and divide it by two—

that's the number of ounces you need each day. But the amount can change. When the weather is warm, for example, you may need more fluid, especially if you are outdoors a lot.

Consider this: if you're ever in your kitchen at eleven o'clock at night and really want something but are not sure what, you're probably thirsty. Pour yourself a glass of something calorie-free and good to drink. Go do something else while you drink it, and you may be fine. When you have problems with food, there may be times when you think you're hungry, when really, you're simply thirsty.

2. **Eat within two hours of rising; eat every three to five hours after that**. If you have problems with food, eating, or weight, and especially if you call yourself a compulsive eater or a food addict, your body needs a regular supply of nutrients to keep the neurotransmitters in your brain balanced and your energy level steady. Plan your schedule to allow time for meals and snacks throughout the day. If the work you are doing is very important to you, you will need every one of your brain cells up, running, and ready to go.

Think about it: how many times when you are dieting have you gone six and eight hours without eating; how many times when bingeing, have you paced your consumption around the addiction's preferences rather than your body's needs? How many times have you skipped a regular meal, planning to indulge yourself later?

If you get up around six a.m., you need to make time to eat breakfast by eight a.m. If you eat breakfast at eight a.m., your next meal should be between eleven a.m. and one p.m. Let's say lunch is at noon. If supper is going to be at five p.m., that's fine, but if you're planning to sit down at the table at seven p.m., you may need a midafternoon snack.

Spreading food consumption this way can be a problem for some, particularly in the beginning. Because when you start eating more frequently, you start thinking about food more frequently too. "Every couple of hours," says my client, "here we go again. It just seems like I'm never not thinking about eating." Yes, that's true. But if you don't eat frequently enough, you allow yourself to get really hungry, which leads to eating too much at the next meal. When you are eating your drug and trigger foods, you are probably thinking about eating all the time. When you stop eating your drug and trigger foods and get through withdrawal (which we'll discuss in another chapter), you won't have that constant urge to eat.

Again, you may be wondering when exactly you should be eating. When you are abstinent (what the next step entails), you should begin to feel hungry ten to fifteen minutes before your next meal or snack and be satisfied when you are done. When you're done with your lunch, you should feel comfortable and satisfied. And whatever time you next get moderately hungry, you should plan to eat within ten to fifteen minutes.

Now, how do you know if it's enough? That's a bit trickier. During recovery, you must learn to really listen to your own inner core of wisdom. Often, when people first put down their binge and drug foods, their whole sense of hunger and fullness disappears. They'll often need someone to tell them the right amount.

> **The only problem with intuitive eating is the body has been so confused by your irregular eating behaviors that it's lost the ability to accurately say what it needs.**

This is a good time to mention that the body is the basis of intuitive eating. The only problem with intuitive eating is the body has been so confused by your irregular eating behaviors that it's lost the ability to accurately say what it needs. The physical changes we have described—the changes in your neurons and neurotransmitters—prevent it from giving you an honest message. It's like asking a drunk to tell you how to get sober. It's not going to work.

A snack, the thing chronic dieters try to cut out of their lives immediately, may be the very thing that allows you to stay on track. A snack is often called a "Metabolic Adjustment." It's a weighed and measured amount of food designed to carry the body from one meal to the next. Food addicts are highly sensitive to changes in their blood sugars. The goal is to keep your blood sugars steady all day long—to avoid wide swings, keep you from getting ravenous between meals, and keep your mood stable enough that you can make healthy decisions.

Also, it's important to provide calories at the time of day your body needs and wants them: to provide energy before exercise; to give you something to eat when everyone around you is snacking; to provide a lift at the time of day you most feel like eating foods that do not serve you.

3. **Eat at least two foods each time you eat, and one should be protein, milk, or yogurt.** Give your body a mixture of protein, fat, and carbohydrates at each meal or snack. Do not eat carbohydrate-containing foods without protein and fat to balance them.

It is paramount that you have protein every time you have carbohydrates. Protein slows down the absorption of carbohydrates and smooths your blood sugar swings.

To break it down into the simplest of terms, here's how I explained these macro (and micro) nutrients to the preschoolers who attended my children's Montessori school: protein is the bricks your body uses to make your muscles and your organs and your nerves and your brain cells. Fat is the mortar between the bricks; it keeps the bricks from hurting each other and scratching at each other. Carbohydrates are the little men in white overalls who lay the bricks. And the vitamins and minerals are the tools and shovels the little men in white overalls use to lay the bricks. So, if you don't have enough iron, the body can't lay the bricks. Iron is the center of the red blood cell—you must put it right in the middle; if you don't, the red blood cell won't work right.

The moral of this story: nutrients need to work together. Please do not eat fruit or carbohydrate all by itself; this may make you hungrier and stir cravings about an hour later. *Your Personal Food Plan Guide* can help. You'll find information at the back of this book.

> **The moral of this story: nutrients need to work together.**

4. **Choose whole foods, real foods, and unrefined foods** in preference to refined, processed, or man-made foods. A man-made food is one that did not exist until man built a factory in which to produce it. The body is a living organism and needs the nutrients of whole food, as close as possible to the way Mother Nature planned them. If you have food and eating problems, the foods you are most likely to be sensitive to are those that are refined, over-processed, or man-made.

5. **Increase to two fruit servings (twelve ounces, total) and two vegetable servings a day.** Choose fruit fresh or frozen, without sugar added. Enjoy it with meals or with a fat-containing dairy or protein as a snack. Vegetables are the most disliked, maligned, misunderstood, and badly prepared foods in our diets. Eat them fresh or frozen, cooked or raw, but learn to prepare and season them effectively, so you can really enjoy them.

Follow these rules for three days to three weeks, until you can do them comfortably and effectively. Whatever else you eat, follow these rules as well. Why, you ask? Because you need to nourish the body and stabilize the neurotransmitters in your brain. When you begin to set aside the foods that harm you, you may feel deprived or unsure of what to eat. Adding these five behaviors will put volume and nutrients into your system; it will make you feel more stable and grounded; and it will force you to look at the healthy, nutrient-rich foods you enjoy from a new perspective.

Important Distinction

Notice I haven't told you to stop eating ice cream at three in the morning. If you drink eight cups of liquid a day and eat half a gallon of ice cream at three in the morning, that's okay for now. When you're deep in the food, you won't be able to take out the problematic stuff from your diet.

Between now and next week, can you just drink eight cups of water a day? I imagine you'd feel guilty if you didn't do something as simple as that, especially when you understand why you need that much water. You do not need to do anything else with your food; just drink that water. Surely, that's attainable.

Then when you get out of bed, eat within two hours. Don't tell yourself that you binged last night, therefore, you're going to starve yourself today. Eat. At eight in the morning . . . and at noon . . . and at five or six . . . and at ten p.m., before you go to bed. Even if you eat hot dogs and French fries, that's better than skipping a meal.

This gives you a pattern to your day. It gives you a way of saying, "Okay, this is the time for my next meal. I'm not starving myself anymore. I'm giving myself food every three to five hours." These meals have protein and fat, which are the most satisfying foods. Your body will feel safe when you do this.

What do I mean by safe? When you eat candy, cake, pie, cookies, the sweet gooey stuff, you introduce a lot of sugar into the body. When absorbed, it goes in quickly. In response, the body makes insulin, more so if you are a food addict. So, if you eat protein and fat with the sugar, your blood sugar will go up, but not as far and not as fast as it would alone. You're going to have more control over what you eat when you need to eat again. So, eat one Entenmann's donut and the body feels frightened; eat twelve, and the body is terrified. But if you eat two mozzarella cheese sticks and a piece of fresh fruit with a doughnut, you're going to feel a lot fuller; maybe the body will feel less frightened; and instead of eating twelve doughnuts, maybe you'll only eat four.

The purpose of this step is to give you a home base. To give you a place to go back to when you have made mistakes. If you can follow this, you will likely be able to keep eating your sane food no matter what else you eat and come back to your sane food plan without a lot of difficulty. Slowly let this become your goal, and it may help you let go of the foods that harm you.

Gifts

Food and eating are precious gifts to our bodies, minds, and spirits. In our journey into insane food behavior, we have lost the ability to recognize the true purpose of this gift. Recovery from food addiction means that we are in the process of rediscovering how to use food to nourish us, and to treat the body with dignity and respect. As we emerge from our addictive behaviors, we begin to recognize and respect the true nature and intention of food – to nourish the body, fuel the mind, and soothe the spirit.

Chapter 6

The Sane Food Eating Plan

Most food plans—okay, let's call them what they are, diets—feel like a straitjacket or a pair of strappy sandals with four-inch heels that hurt your feet. But a food plan should feel like a comfortable old sweater or your favorite pair of sneakers.

What's so special about your favorite pair of sneakers? They're warm; they support you well; when you slog through mud or hike up a hill, they help keep you balanced; they keep you moving forward. Your food plan should do the same. If you get a blister from a new pair of shoes, you change the shoes, you don't cut off your toe. Likewise, if your food plan pinches or restricts you, if it leaves you hungry or overfull, change the food plan. Your food plan should be safe enough, comfortable enough, and supportive enough to carry you safely through your rocky path of food recovery.

A food plan that is comfortable for your abstinence:

- Takes out your binge, drug, trigger foods, and your destructive behaviors.
- Meets the body's nutrient needs while moving the body toward a normal weight.

- Is enough; ensures you feel satisfied.
- Allows you to feel your feelings. (Don't worry. This will be explained.)
- Gives you space for creating the mental, emotional, and spiritual recovery you want.

First Things First

The next step is to remove your binge, trigger, and drug foods. Since the issue you've been having with food is a physiological, biochemical uniqueness in your body, it is essential for you to remove the foods that are causing a physical reaction.

> **Since the issue you've been having with food is a physiological, biochemical uniqueness in your body, it is essential for you to remove the foods that are causing a physical reaction.**

A trigger food, as we've established, is a food that sets off the binge process. I recommend you take out all the foods you binge on; then take a hard look at the foods that are like those foods. Once you take out the foods that cause a physical reaction, the cravings will fade.

As I've said before, the kinds and amounts of foods needed to induce a physical reaction are different for everyone. For some, even the tiniest amount of food can cause a reaction because it releases neurotransmitters in your brain that smooth out your feelings. The minute a foreign substance enters the body, it has a reaction. That's why alcoholics must avoid all foods that contain alcohol, even flavorings.

Of course, one of your challenges will be the need to listen to your body differently and adjust to what it's telling you. If you are under a lot of stress, you may find that your threshold for these substances is lower, requiring you to be more careful—not more indulgent—when you are under stress. Abstinence boundaries can help.

Food and Feeling Boundaries

In recovery, a boundary is a line you draw between you and certain foods and behaviors. There are different kinds of boundaries: some foods need to be excluded from your plate because they have proven themselves to cause difficulties for you; some you'll only eat at certain times or in special situations; some need to be included in your food plan every day for the health and well-being of your body.

Barbed Wire Boundaries

Barbed wire boundaries protect you from your binge and drug foods. I call them red areas. You never go beyond them; that way you stay safe. Cross them and you've gone too far; you're in trouble, no longer in abstinence, and back to the pendulum swinging.

This is how you cut from your food plan those foods and behaviors that always give you trouble—including the foods that come with them, or that look and act like them, as well as the behaviors associated with them. Keep them out no matter what. If you find yourself in a red area, please, sit down and call for help!

Yellow Areas

Yellow areas are dangerous trigger foods. They never include your addictive foods or behaviors, but they still make you forget yourself. So, you only go there when absolutely necessary.

Sometimes life gets screwy, and you need to move away from your usual boundaries for a special situation: you're in the emergency room with a family member at two a.m.; you're backpacking in Israel, on a transatlantic flight, sick and throwing up; you're preparing for a medical procedure. In such situations, you may need a meal or snack you don't usually have. Be careful in such times. Ask for help from people you can trust. After these situations are resolved, you may go back to your regular food plan; you may even choose to use a bit more structure or be more careful for a while.

Green Areas

As you might gather, green areas are the foods, nutrients, and behaviors that are comfortable, safe, and satisfying for you. They work because they're right for your body and right for your life. They're comfortable and easy—more like a sweatshirt than a straitjacket. Within your plan, this is the way you live and eat nearly 100% of the time. You have room to move, to live, within your abstinence boundaries. These are the foods we will discuss next.

The Sane Food Plan

When you look at abstinence from self-abuse with food, you want it to be nutrient-rich, not simply free of drug, trigger, and binge foods. You must give your body all the nutrients it needs at the time of day it needs them most. This means high-quality nutrient-rich foods with lots of calcium and B vitamins and reasonable amounts of healthy fats and the nutrients your body best uses to repair, replace, and restore itself. The way you eat has a major effect on the structure and function of your body; you need to repair the damage your abusive eating behaviors created.

Most of the time, diets don't give you enough nutrients to allow the body to maintain its structure and function adequately. That's one of the reasons you keep struggling against yourself. If you're hungry, you will struggle. If you have too few nutrients or the food plan is not balanced for you, you will have a hard time overriding the body's urges. Again, physiology is stronger than willpower 99.999% of the time. For now, these guidelines will help as you inch your way to recovery.

> **Physiology is stronger than willpower 99.999% of the time.**

Basic Guidelines

1. The body needs fluids.

I won't reiterate what I said about hydration in the last chapter, but I do want to emphasize one fact: dehydration is the only illness that can reliably kill you within three days. Again, there are different recommendations about the amount you need to drink: eight cups (sixty-four ounces) a day; take your body weight in pounds, divide it by two, and drink that many fluid ounces a day. This works well even though it seems like a lot. Don't use coffee, diet soda, or other artificially sweetened beverages for this fluid allowance; instead, choose water, seltzer, herbal tea, or hot or iced tea instead.

2. The body needs to be fed every three to five hours while you are awake.

You may need to change your eating schedule to allow this, but it is so very important! If you let yourself go longer than five hours without eating, you may find yourself ravenous at the next meal or snack and eat much more than you intended. By now, you've probably seen how eating often enough keeps you from bingeing when you're hungry.

3. **Focus on meeting the body's nutrient needs.**

Your body's nutrient needs partly depend on your body height, weight, and size, your activity level, and your nutrition status. Again, opinions vary, but here is a general list:

- Fruits: two to four servings a day (a serving is a single piece of fruit, or about six ounces)
- Vegetables, raw, cooked, or a mixture: three to five cups a day
- Protein from meat, cheese, beans, fish, or other sources: six to twelve ounces a day
- Fats, no trans-fat, and using mostly unsaturated fats: two to six tablespoons a day
- Cereals, starches, and grains (preferably whole grains): three to twelve servings a day, only the ones you can tolerate and without added sugars
- Milk and milk products (or some other calcium source): two to three servings a day

When you put together your plan, allow for some protein or milk/yogurt at each meal/snack. You will notice that each of your meals and snacks will have protein or milk/yogurt in them. You can customize the serving amounts to match your needs.

Women need 1,000-1,200 milligrams of calcium a day. That equals two to three cups of milk or yogurt. If you're unwilling or unable to meet your needs for calcium with milk or yogurt, you may substitute calcium fortified soy milk, or choose to take calcium supplements instead.

All people need protein to maintain muscle mass and organ tissue. Protein is essential for the body's structure and function as well as the building blocks for hormones, blood, and bone. For protein you need a piece of meat approximately the size of the palm of your hand and about as thick as the side of your hand, twice a day. Or you need the equivalent in other protein sources. People with food addiction often need more protein or fat than others. This is, again, to control the rate of food absorption and maintain stable blood sugars.

4. **Make sure to provide the calories at the time of day the body needs them.**

Starving all day, then eating a lot before bedtime only gives the body more work and less time to rest. Eating all your calories at one time only prolongs hunger and the body's "I must save calories" response. Starving your body is like a diet. It will lead to weight gain at the end of the starvation period—and your body has had enough of that (which I'll get into later).

Decide now the most effective timing of your meals and metabolics (smaller meal-like food choices). At which meal do you need the most calories; are you the hungriest? Which meal corresponds to the time of day you need your body and mind to be functioning at their best? This is the meal that should be your largest meal.

What if you need your body and mind to function best around more than one meal (as is consistent with much of the American lifestyle)—what then? When do you go six or eight hours without food? Should you put a snack in? Do you need something at bedtime; will it let you sleep better, or will it start a binge? Is there a time of day when you cannot seem to eat appropriately? Examine this time closely; what is it you really need—a nap, a friend, or some more helpful foods?

You need to consider all these and more when spreading out your food during the day to meet your particular needs.

5. **Eat appropriate foods you enjoy.**

At the start of this new journey, you've been eating protein at each meal and a little fat to offset the blood sugar spike that accompanies carbohydrate consumption. While this is important, you do not need to eat boring diet food all day. Find new foods you like; try new recipes and new spices and seasonings and begin to enjoy your meals. Food should be pleasurable, even when it is devoid of the substances your addiction craves.

6. **Listen to your body and treat the body with respect.**

Take time to take care of your body so it can take care of you. The body is a gift to the mind and spirit, for learning and growth; learn the lessons of a healthy body. Speak kindly to it.

The body has several goals. The first goal is your survival; the body will do whatever it takes to ensure you survive. If you don't get enough calcium in your food, the body will take calcium from your bones to keep your heart beating because a beating heart is more important than strong bones. If you try to take out all the fat in your diet, your body becomes terrified because the body feels like it is going to starve to death. So, you must respect your body by providing it with all the nutrients it needs to maintain itself.

And if your mind is clouded by addictive agents that interfere with your neurotransmitters, it cannot best serve the body's needs. When you do good things for the body, you think more clearly.

Talk With a Trusted Friend or Professional

We all need help sometimes. Find people you can trust who care about you. Let them help you. This group of trusted advisors may be outside of your usual supporters, since friends and family may be eating nearly as badly as you are.

I'm touching on this now (we'll discuss further in Chapter 10) because setting up your meal plan may be one of the first areas where you need support. It's change, and change can be frightening, not to mention, there are a lot of things to consider. A dietitian or nutritionist, a sponsor or a trusted friend can help. The key is to choose someone who knows a lot about food, eating, and body weight, and your chosen recovery path.

In my office, I used to write food plans in pencil on paper to demonstrate that it is not carved in stone. Now, of course, I use a computer program because so many live far away and it's faster and easier, and more user friendly. Still, the fact remains. To the best of my knowledge, Moses did not come down off the mountain with a food plan. Food plans are an estimate of a guesstimate of an average. Even though I calculate and write individual food plans for each client, tailored to their preferences, body, and needs, there may still be adjustments.

That's why support is important. And it can be extremely valuable to talk with a dietitian/nutritionist who is familiar with the Twelve Step principles. Then, you can apply the principles learned here, work with your trusted adviser on it, work through recovery issues, change as you need to, and come to the point of enjoying your food and your recovery.

> **It can be extremely valuable to talk with a dietitian/nutritionist who is familiar with the Twelve Step principles.**

Your Personal Food Plan Guide can help. You'll find information on this at the back of this book.

Writing Your Food Plan

Before you create your food plan, based on your particular needs, it may be a good idea to know what one looks like. Here's a sample. This plan is very much like the one used by Glenbeigh Hospital of Tampa, Florida, which had the first food addiction rehab unit in the late 1980s. Many of the other food plans you see in recovery circles are similar to this one.

<u>*Breakfast*</u>
6 oz. fruit
1 oz. cereal or ½ cup starch
2 eggs (2 oz. protein)
8 oz. low-fat milk or yogurt

<u>*Lunch*</u>
3 oz. protein equivalent
4 oz. potato or 3 oz. starch
6–8 oz. vegetables, raw or cooked or both
2 Tbsp. oil or any other fat to total 28–32 grams fat
6 oz. fruit

<u>*Dinner*</u>
3 oz. protein equivalent
4 oz. potato or 3 oz. starch
6–8 oz. vegetables, raw or cooked or both
2 Tbsp. oil or fat to total 28–32 g. fat

<u>Bed</u>

6 oz. fruit

1 oz. cereal

8 oz. low-fat milk or yogurt

**Notice please! This is only an example. Your food needs may be very different. You will need to adjust for the needs of your unique body, using basic healthy food principles. Working with a professional can help you fine tune a food plan so that it fits you just right. Also notice, there is a specific measurement associated with these menu items. We will discuss the importance of measuring and weighing your food in Chapter 9: Daily Practices.

Metabolic Adjustments

Food plans include smaller meal-like food choices. By now you should have incorporated these into your day to keep hunger at bay. You'll find a list of suggestions for these foods in the bonus materials located here: www.sanefood.com/bonus/. These suggestions all include more than one food; they have some sources of fat and carbohydrate and protein (such as meat, eggs, milk, cheese, yogurt, or a vegetarian protein) because we want to keep your nutrients balanced and avoid eating large amounts of a particular food.

Don't eat fruit all by itself or in more than one portion. All the calories in fruit come from a simple carbohydrate named fructose; if there's not enough protein to balance that fructose, you can increase the amount and intensity of your cravings. Fructose is absorbed from your intestines and sent to the liver to be converted to glucose. The glucose is released into the bloodstream about an hour after eating fruit, and that is when you would likely feel hungry or have more cravings. So, always include protein. For example, six ounces of fruit and two ounces of protein would look like two cheese sticks and a cup of blueberries, or two tablespoons of peanut butter and an apple, or half a cup of cottage cheese and a cup of pineapple.

As stated before, knowing how much food to include will not be easy. It's one of the parts of recovery that teaches you to really listen to your own inner core of wisdom. I help calculate the right amount for my clients; it's one more reason you don't want to do this alone.

The Spirit in Which to Write Your Food Plan

Following the general guidelines provided, write your food plan—gently, carefully, quietly. You are walking on sacred ground . . .

> **Following the general guidelines provided, write your food plan—gently, carefully, quietly. You are walking on sacred ground . . .**

You may have been told things that hurt you. Friends, family, coaches, programs—they may have told you things that are not true for you. Because of their authority, you pretended to believe them. You did what they said, and it did not work. Then they blamed you. They said you did not do it right. You had no willpower. They called you lazy, weak, unable to follow instructions. You felt beaten . . . ashamed, incompetent, worthless . . . a failure. And they took lots of your money, time, and faith.

But I'm here to tell you that this is not your fault. You did not cause it. You did not create it. It can be fixed.

Listen carefully to what you are feeling, what has been happening. Ask questions about your body, about your life, about what you like. Look for what you want and need—what works for you. Ask your Higher Power to guide you and listen for the response.

Don't be afraid to ask for help. If you need someone to break out the calculator and calculate the calories you need now for your goal weight, and maybe a weight in between, ask one of your trusted advisers. Together you can calculate your protein needs, your fat needs, and your other nutrient needs—vitamins, minerals, calcium, fluid.

As you write, be sure to incorporate your unique comfort and lifestyle, nutritional and medical requirements, and cut opportunities for wrong food choices to sneak in. Try one of the plans in *Your Personal Food Plan Guide*. (Again, you'll find more information at the back of this book.)

Your food plan should fit your body, mind, and heart. It should always be leading you toward your goals. As you write, ask yourself, "How does this feel?" Make changes if needed; enjoy if it fits you well.

Timing the Meals to Fit Your Needs

Again, customization is essential because no two people share the same requirements. Our lives are too different for a one-size-fits-all meal plan, even though the latest diet may claim otherwise. As you know, it's not simply what you do or do not eat, but also when you eat. This, too, must be personalized. Here are a few examples:

Sally gets up at 5:45 every morning. She goes to the gym for an hour, then comes home, gets dressed, and goes to work from 8:30 a.m. to 4:30 p.m. She goes to bed between 9:30 and 10 p.m.

Her meal plan: metabolic at 6 a.m.; breakfast at 7:30 a.m.; lunch at noon; perhaps she will have a metabolic at 4 p.m. and dinner at 6:30 p.m.—or maybe she won't want a midafternoon food time; she will just have dinner at 5:30 or 6 p.m. and be in bed by 9:30 p.m. (She is 38 years old, 5'6" and weighs 200 pounds. Her goal is to lose 1 to 1 ½ pounds a week.)

Suzie is a bank teller. She has two children at home. She works from 8 a.m. to 4 p.m. (sometimes 6 p.m.). She eats breakfast at 7 a.m. and lunch at 11:30 a.m. She needs a snack at 3 or 4 p.m.; then it's home, homework, and dinner at 6 or 7 p.m. She is up till 11 p.m., so she needs a bedtime metabolic at 9:30 or 10 p.m. (She also is 38, 5'6" and weighs 130. Her goal is to maintain her weight.)

Sylvia is retired. She has breakfast whenever she rises, then lunch at noon or 1 p.m. Her dinner is early, at 5 or 6 p.m.. She does not want a bedtime metabolic; "Leave me alone after dinner, dear; I go to bed early most nights." (She is 72, 5'4" and weighs 135 pounds. Her goal is lots of nutrients and enough energy.)

Steve is a construction worker. He needs to be at work by 6 a.m. and finishes work at 2:30 p.m. or so. His request, "Don't make me eat those girlie foods!" He needs breakfast very early (at 5 a.m. or so); lunch is packed in his lunchbox and eaten with the guys promptly at 11:30 a.m. When he gets home, he is ravenous. He will have a large metabolic after work, then dinner with his family at 6:30 p.m. or so. He goes to bed by 9 p.m., so he does not want any food at bedtime. His meals will seem huge because he is very active and needs a lot of calories during the day. (Steve is 6'2" and weighs 240 pounds; this will maintain his weight.)

We have said that the food plan is to become the core of your recovery process. What will that mean? It means that it will be the center point around which you will build your recovery program. It has to fit you perfectly. Like a deeply loved pair of sneakers, it has to support you in the places you need support, give you freedom to move and work and live your life, and keep you from getting tripped up by the messiness of the food world around you. It is absolutely essen-

> **It is absolutely essential to have a food plan that fits *your* body and your needs.**

tial to have a food plan that fits *your* body and *your* needs. It should not make you feel deprived or regimented, rather supported and protected. It should become a real comfort space in your life, which will make it much easier to follow and work with.

Now, to make it work for you. Think about your daily life and your usual schedule. What hours does your body need to eat; what hours will your schedule permit you to eat? This is tough. Pick your most common day first. Go down into your heart of hearts and look at what you really need: what time of day does your body really want food; when can you fit regular meals comfortably? Then, start your sleeping time (seven to eight hours a night, please); add work and travel time. Fill in your mealtimes.

Considerations

Another piece of the timing puzzle revolves around your unique situation. Say you have your lunch at noon and usually get to dinner at eight o'clock; you will need a larger snack in the afternoon than if you usually get to dinner at six or six-thirty. This is what it means to allow enough food for fullness and comfort.

You need to consider any medical conditions. Are there foods you can't eat or foods you need to eat more or less of to manage your medical issues; are there changes you should make to handle your medical conditions more effectively?

Then there are your trigger situations. Consider when you eat the foods you later regret—and why. I've said it before; willpower won't help. Physiology will trump willpower every day of the week. What time do you most often find yourself going off into an eating nightmare: is it four p.m. when you get home from work, need to make dinner, and help with your children's activities and homework; is it during the day when your boss or customers annoy you? Do you avoid overeating all day, waiting for that special time when everyone is settled, so you can be alone with the food, or do you wake up in the middle of the night to eat your fill in private? (Don't feel bad; many of my clients do.)

Follow your food plan for a few weeks so you have some experience with how well (or poorly) the timing works for you.

> ### EXERCISE: Determine (and adjust) your meal timing

- What time is your breakfast, and is it a main meal of your day?
- Do you need more food? Less food?
- Do you exercise first thing in the morning? If so, do you need a small exercise supplement in addition to or instead of part of breakfast and breakfast after exercise?
- What is your morning like? Is it long and unpredictable?
- Do you need the second half of breakfast, or an additional amount of food, to make it to lunch?
- How does lunch fit? Do you need more or less of something?
- How long is it from lunch to supper? Do you need an extra supplement?
- If this time is too long and you wind up ravenous and bingeing at dinnertime, do you need a measured amount of food at 3 or 4 p.m. (and will you still be able to enjoy your dinner)?

- How are the amounts at dinnertime: enough; too much; too little?
- Add bedtime food. Most of us want something comforting before bed. What do you need to have that will not start a binge?
- Look carefully and change what does not work for you. Will you be satisfied with the plan you have created?
- Are your binge opportunities gone? Are you meeting your needs for calcium, B vitamins, and minerals? Are you meeting your other needs?

Adjust and try this food plan for two weeks and see what happens. Talk to a sponsor or trusted person every day and look carefully at what is working; change what is not working. Try again.

Keep going till you have a food plan that meets your needs—physically, mentally, emotionally, and spiritually. One that keeps you from food abuse and allows you to concentrate on a recovery program.

This is self-care with food. This is your plan, and no one else's. It needs to fit you and meet your needs. Yes, I am asking you to set aside (or kick to the curb) all the drug and binge foods and the foods you think you don't want to be without. Trust me on this. If you leave them out for a while, they will be there and ready for you if this doesn't work. But they will bring you the same consequences that they had before.

What is Sane Food?

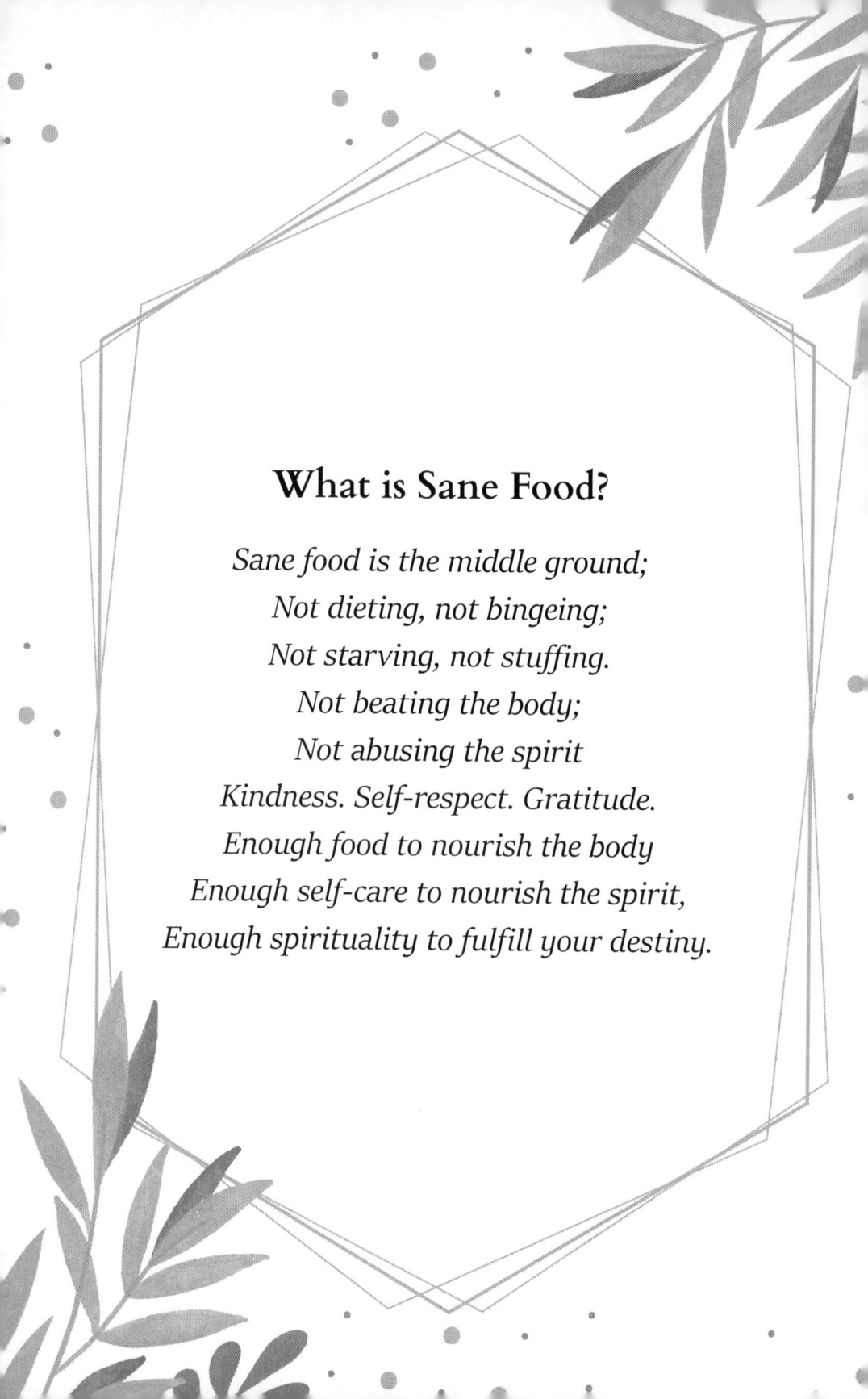

*Sane food is the middle ground;
Not dieting, not bingeing;
Not starving, not stuffing.
Not beating the body;
Not abusing the spirit
Kindness. Self-respect. Gratitude.
Enough food to nourish the body
Enough self-care to nourish the spirit,
Enough spirituality to fulfill your destiny.*

Chapter 7

Withdrawal, Cravings, and Triggers

The five hallmarks of any physical addiction are tolerance, cravings, physical withdrawal, obsessions, and loss of control. We see all of these in food addiction. You developed tolerance when you needed more and more of your drug food to get the same result. Now that you've removed these foods, you need to be aware of the specific withdrawal symptoms, both physical and emotional, that occur, so you can safeguard your recovery.

Once you remove the drug, trigger, and binge foods from your plate, you will start having feelings. These are the feelings you may have been pushing down with food. By the third day, you will likely find yourself wanting to eat everything you can get your hands on. You will experience strong cravings for high-nutrient or low-nutrient food. The first things you may notice now that you're practicing abstinence (though you may not associate them with a change in what you're eating) are the symptoms of withdrawal.

> **The five hallmarks of any physical addiction are tolerance, cravings, physical withdrawal, obsessions, and loss of control.**

Withdrawal

Withdrawal is the pain you feel when you stop using the food items to which the body is sensitive or addicted. Part of the withdrawal is due to the physical changes that have occurred in your body; part is due to the loss of your primary coping skill; part is related to the many lifestyle changes you need to make in recovery.

Physical withdrawal occurs in stages. The primary and most severe stage occurs in the first five days of eating abstinently; we suspect the other stages may last months or even years into recovery.

Common withdrawal symptoms that may occur well into recovery include:

- Inability to think clearly; "brain fog" or feeling "fuzzy"
- Short- or long-term memory lapses
- Feelings of grief
- Emotional lability
- Numbness
- Sleep disturbances
- Periods of overwhelming anger
- Irrational fears
- Oversensitivity to stress
- Problems with coordination

Withdrawal symptoms require support. You cannot fully recover from addiction on your own because many of the arising emotions will drive you back to food.

You may not like it; you may even hate it, but you will also experience triggers and cravings. Physical cravings are part of withdrawal symptoms; they can last intermittently for three months or more. They will happen at some point in your recovery. Accept this.

Remember, acceptance is not approval; it's putting a stop to resisting reality. If you missed it the first time, don't worry, I'll say it again.

Cravings

A craving for alcohol is normal for an alcoholic. A craving for a slot machine is normal for a gambler. A craving for a drug food is normal for a food addict. It's a message from your body, mind, or spirit that something is off kilter. Heed the message: take care of the real problem; don't medicate with food or other methods. Over time, cravings will become helpful parts of your life, making you aware of the matters that need your attention and giving you the opportunity to focus on the next step in your recovery.

In your recovery process, your brain will start calling for specific foods—not your stomach, your brain. This is a craving. It's the urge to eat, do, or use a food or other drug in an abusive or self-destructive way; it's a nagging, under the surface, persistent thought about a food. It may be to escape a feeling or be full. Or it may be an actual, clear thought: "I need to eat; feel normal; not feel deprived."

The desire often feels uncontrollable, irresistible, and never-ending. A client once told me, "I'd been craving them desperately for days, so I decided to just go eat them and get it over with." Another described it as very intense and all encompassing: "If I were on a plane heading straight down, it would be, 'Yes, I know we are heading for a crash! I'll fix it; just let me eat this first!'"

A craving can come out of nowhere and feel like a ton of bricks fell on you. Yet another client described it this way: "It is a driving force that overtakes my brain. I can think of nothing else. It involves all of my consciousness, and my brain is on autopilot. I feel like I will die if I don't get that food." Then there's this: "When I need to eat, it's like if you took a whole box of Ex-Lax and tried to not go to the bathroom for forty-eight hours. Impossible. Overwhelming. Irresistible."

Every person experiences cravings differently. Cravings are nearly always for the food you know you should not eat. Often the craving is for a processed food that is not healthy or nutritious, and it may be a food you have eaten abusively in the past. Even though the conscious mind sees these foods as unhealthy and not helpful choices, some other part of the brain disagrees and wants them. This is not about a lack of willpower; it goes much more deeply than that. For some, overprocessed and refined foods stimulate the reward system in the brain the same way addictive drugs (like cocaine) do. In some people, this can lead to a full-blown addictive process.

I believe cravings that feel physical, emotional, or spiritual are proof positive that a physical change, adjustment, or response is happening in the body. It's not your choice. It's your addiction. And this proves your physical sensitivity and need to continue this process.

You may recall, the brain and body's primary goal is survival. The positive reward system is set up to activate whenever you do something that promotes survival, like eating food that tastes good. The brain releases dopamine and other feel-good chemicals into the reward system. The problem with modern man-made foods is that they can cause a reward that feels way more powerful than any whole food. So, while the dopamine released by a luscious steak dinner is rewarding, the dessert causes the most powerful dopamine surge. This encourages susceptible people to eat overprocessed and refined foods more often and in larger amounts.

Yes, cravings often have a physical component because of the way our brains are wired, but they also have an emotional and spiritual component as well, including:

- Maladaptive thoughts
- Unresolved feelings
- Spiritual issues

This is why your cravings can become vital parts of your recovery process—they can give you all sorts of information about yourself: how your day is going; what you're feeling; what's going on in your recovery life; how to handle a relationship issue. It's important that you learn to hear the message a craving has to give, to understand and use that information, and to cope with the cravings themselves.

You do not have to let cravings rule your life. Using your recovery tools, you can learn to tolerate the temporary discomfort of a craving and redirect it. Whenever you do this, your sense of self control will increase and strengthen, and it will be easier to handle a craving the next time.

Always remember a craving is like a wave on the ocean; it has a beginning, it crests, and then it subsides. A craving will always subside if you do not empower it. A craving will not last longer than three minutes unless you entertain it. A craving will only get stronger if you feed it.

> **A craving will always subside if you do not empower it.**

The Four Types of Cravings

Cravings are linked to many things: you didn't eat all your food or the right food at your last meal; it's time to eat your next meal; you're having a feeling; you're in a situation you used to eat over. It could also be that you ate something you're sensitive to at your last meal.

Cravings can be roughly divided into four types, based on their source: physical, mental, emotional, and spiritual. Usually, they are not a product of the body but the brain, specifically in the regions of the brain that are responsible for memory, pleasure, and reward. An imbalance of hormones, such as leptin and serotonin, can cause food cravings. Sometimes they are due to endorphins that are released into the body after one has eaten. Most often, they are a mental response to unpleasant feelings or memories, or the need for comfort.

Let's talk about each type in turn . . .

Physical Cravings

Cravings can sometimes originate in the body. This can be due to a lack of fluids or to a deficiency in certain nutrients. A physical craving comes from a physical error. The body needs or thinks it needs more food or a different kind of food.

If you have eaten a food to which you are sensitive, you may notice cravings for three to five days. And when you first stop eating foods to which you are sensitive, you will feel urgent pushes to eat your drug food again. The absence of the drug food causes pain in the neurotransmitters in the brain. The brain can actually create the sense of pain and urgency to return itself to normal. Are you eating some questionable foods that may be triggering you? This is so important. If there is a new food or a questionable food in your diet, the first symptom of physical intolerance is cravings.

Hunger and thirst can produce very similar sensations in the mind, causing it to become confused. One of the easiest ways to reduce food cravings is to make sure the body is hydrated throughout the day. So, get a bottle of water or a cup of tea.

Stress may cause cravings on its own. It results in higher levels of cortisol, the stress hormone, which may promote your cravings. How stressed are you? Maybe you need more self-care.

Many studies have shown that not getting enough sleep could alter the body's hormonal balance. This imbalance contributes to your cravings.

Under-eating can also make food cravings worse. Are you eating enough; are you getting all your protein and fat? A healthy diet does not include frequent hunger pangs. In fact, when the body is very hungry, it may crave more calorie-dense foods than usual, including fried and processed foods. Often people with eating disorders restrict foods, especially fats, when they are trying to control their eating. The body then becomes hungry, and the physical hunger combines with the cravings to create a sense of urgency for eating.

What to do in response to a physical craving:

If you start craving something, take a deep breath. Call someone you trust if you can. Ask your Higher Power to send help and wisdom. Get some ice water or some hot tea; maybe grab a good book, your knitting, or your favorite magazine. Allow yourself a good cry if that's what's needed.

Changing habits is hard work. Your old eating habits will try to come back for a long time. Start new habits to replace them. If you have a craving, handle it right away.

These items all help safeguard your food plan:

- Don't skip meals. Eat healthy food every three to five hours.

- Eat all the food on your food plan. Be especially careful to get all the fat servings.

- Eat on a regular schedule. Try not to have big differences in the timing of meals.

- Are you having little bites of drug foods? These tiny excursions may cause increased cravings.

- If postponing a meal is necessary, then add or move one of your smaller meals to cover the time without food. If you unexpectedly have a delayed meal, eat that meal and the next meal on your usual schedule, or as soon as you are ready for it. Expect to feel hungrier for the next meal and for a few hours afterwards.

- If you have not been eating your binge or drug foods for some time, and you begin to have unexplained physical cravings, do a "food audit." In the next twenty-four to forty-eight hours, reread the labels on all the foods you eat. Has the manufacturer changed one of your usual foods? Are you eating an incorrect portion?

- Extra fluids help here, as do extra sleep and appropriate exercise.

Mental Cravings

Your thoughts can cause cravings. If you allow yourself to mentally ruminate on the idea that you can't live without your favorite foods, that you simply won't survive without them, that you can't stand the pain of not having them, then you can increase your cravings by your thoughts. If you spend time thinking about how much you miss a given food, how much you want it, or what it means to you and your life, you increase its presence and power in your life. These are some thoughts that are so habitual they come up nearly without stimulus.

There is an "incentive salience theory" that suggests that your addiction has a place in your subconscious mind. It's an intense kind of wanting; your brain has developed an association between the addictive food and feeling better. Even if you've been abstinent for a long time, this subconscious connection may not fade or may be reactivated under stress. It does not always mean that you are doing anything wrong. The compulsive urgency to get the drug food can seem extremely strong.

What to do with a mental craving:

It's vitally important that you control what you say to yourself. Your mind and body will respond to the directions your brain gives them. So, pay attention to what's going on in your mind: are there thoughts you would have eaten over in the past; are you worrying about something; is your mind racing; are you struggling with disturbing thoughts?

Some of the hardest habits to change are the thoughts in your mind. Many of these thoughts are things you have been told since childhood, they led to your problems with food, and the thoughts help maintain more thoughts. Thoughts lead to actions and vice versa, which is how the cycle persists.

Think about the person you are and the person you want to become. Why are you changing your food? Either a thought supports your new way of living and eating, or you need to change the thought. Confront it. Reject it. Tell it you no longer want to hear that stuff. Then replace it with a thought that reflects your new goals. Create in your mind a positive response, one that leads you to the result you want. For the thoughts of the foods, create a pattern of self-supportive sentences, such as, "I am working on a new way of eating. I'm learning to change my habits. I'm becoming more comfortable with my eating. This time I am getting the help I need to succeed."

Here are some examples of positive affirmations to help you interrupt a negative thought cycle:

- I am choosing to take better care of my body.
- This is my new way of living and eating.
- I am choosing to change my food, eating, and other habits to create the life I want.
- I deserve the life I want. Even if it does not seem possible right now, I choose to become the person I was meant to be and have the life I deserve.
- Through this struggle is where I will grow, and I am grateful for this guidance and experience.
- I want to create a life that makes me happy.
- I am becoming more courageous and willing to take risks for the things I want.
- My life is full of possibilities; I can have or create a life that makes me happy.
- I want to become the woman that God, my Higher Power, or my Inner Core of Wisdom wants me to be. I am determined to move in that direction.
- I am meant to be strong, powerful, joyful, and full of love and life.
- I am worth the love I have and the love that I will have.
- I am learning to appreciate every moment of my life.

Choose from these affirmations or create the ones that express what you want to attract into your life. Make them positive, present tense, and believable. Change them to fit what you really want to create. Set up five of them and post them where you will see them regularly. Now when the negative thoughts come, repeat these sentences instead.

It may sound nutty at first to say these sentences when you are struggling with a food craving, but try it! You'll find it really does help.

Emotional Cravings

Sometimes cravings are the product of memories from the past when you had certain feelings and ate your drug foods immediately. Now, having the feeling leads to food use almost automatically without thinking about it, and often you can't even name or recognize the feeling.

Understand that feelings do not simply go away. They must be felt and heard. Early on in recovery, one feeling may trigger another, then another. The total can be overwhelming. That's because you have been eating your feelings rather than processing them. You need a new program for processing the feelings and a new procedure for handling the situations that trouble you in your life.

> **Understand that feelings do not simply go away. They must be felt and heard.**

What to do in response to emotional cravings:

You may feel like you must do something. One of the simplest responses to this pressure is to pretend the craving came to you in an email you did not expect. In the email, they're telling you that your credit card will be charged $479 for an item you do not remember ordering. Your first question is, "Is this mine; is it something I ordered?" Similarly, with a craving, refuse to eat until you know what the feeling is. If you can't identify the feeling right away, call someone you trust, or try journaling. Especially late at night or when you wake in the middle of the night, make yourself write at least five sentences about what is happening in your life and what you are feeling before you allow yourself to eat inappropriately.

Some feelings come and flow like ocean waves. If it feels so strong that it may overwhelm you, you need only relax and allow it time to ebb. Reassure yourself. This is a feeling. All that a feeling needs from you is that you feel it 100% and hear its message. Then it can leave you.

Know that if you have a good binge you are going to have cravings for more, for forty-eight to seventy-two hours. The most important thing to remember: do not go head-to-head with your cravings. As an old Chinese saying goes, "When you see your enemy coming at you full speed, step aside."

Spiritual Cravings

Eating is the most intimate experience of our lives. Food actually becomes a physical part of the body. So, the longing you feel for food can be a longing for some spiritual connection—for love, hope, support, or comfort, for the presence of a Higher Power. The Twelve Step Program and a whole host of world religions offer great varieties of choices in this area. But spirituality is not the same as religion; it involves the conscious contact with your own inner spiritual self and a sense of who you are in the universe. As you come more deeply into connection with your inner self, your inner core of wisdom, and your Higher Power, you will feel more peaceful and calmer about yourself.

What to do about a spiritual craving:

When you feel that inner longing, use it as a trigger to pray, or meditate, or journal. Sit with whatever spiritual practice helps you, but if your current practice does not help, feel free to change it.

Have you been avoiding your spiritual program or struggling with some spiritual issue? Are you angry with your Higher Power, struggling to believe, or finding it hard to make time for prayer? Ask yourself these questions, and journal it out.

What do you really need: a phone call, meeting, prayer, time alone, a change or comfort in your life? Are you happy and wanting to celebrate; are you in the middle of taking a difficult step? Maybe you're not taking a step that's needed; maybe you had a difficult talk with someone, and it's still in your mind. Maybe you need more support, more friendships, more contact with other people. Maybe you're lonely.

Never indulge a craving by eating it. That will make it stronger and more persistent. Cravings demonstrate the physical nature and power of your food addiction. Instead, let them confirm for you that this is a physical issue, and you are on the right path to freedom.

Emergency Craving Response

When cravings strike, they often come on very strongly; you may have the illusion that the craving is irresistible. Regardless of the type, cravings will go away under one of two circumstances: when you decide to eat, or when you decide that you will not eat, no matter what. If you feel the craving, you also feel a kind of anxiety. Once you decide which path you will take, the anxiety begins to diminish, as will the craving.

Your cravings will not continue to escalate to the point of being intolerable unless you invite them to stay for a cup of tea. That's when you discuss with yourself the merits of eating or not eating the food; debate and tell yourself you really shouldn't; remember how good the food used to taste; how guilty you feel about eating it; on and on it goes. When you entertain cravings this way, it usually means you need more nurturing, more support, or time for yourself—maybe even time for a little play.

The more experience you have with successfully resisting cravings, the easier it becomes. If you have successfully handled cravings in the past, you will prove to yourself that you can handle them again.

> **The more experience you have with successfully resisting cravings, the easier it becomes.**

Refusing a craving is actually quite easy.

First, you label it as a craving. "Yup, that's a craving. I do not need to eat over it. Even though I want to eat this food, even though I wish I could feel the relief of eating it, the world won't stop if I don't."

Second, you make a clear decision. "No. I am not eating this."

Third, you go do something else. Put your mind on any other activity. Do some sudoku. Sing a song. Recite multiplication tables. Say the Serenity Prayer in its five versions, five times. Make a phone call. Read some literature. Journal.

The moment your attention is on something else, is the moment the craving starts to diminish. The more focused you are on the new activity, the more rapidly the craving will go away.

Remind yourself, "This cannot last forever." Remember the times you were not craving. Every time you have a craving is important.

Every time you have a craving, you are given the opp⟨...⟩ strengthen your recovery or to weaken it. Every time matte⟨...⟩ every time makes you stronger or weaker; it teaches you to s⟨...⟩ or to conquer.

> ## EXERCISE: Managing a craving

To manage cravings, you must learn to process them in a way that diminishes their power and enhances your recovery. Do not run and hide or avoid a craving; process it immediately.

Here are some suggestions for handling those moments when a craving has you in its grip:

- Take three deep breaths. Nothing bad will happen. Reassure yourself that you are safe.
- Pause; find a peaceful place in your mind. You will not starve to death in the next five minutes. Notice that you're okay.
- Think about your thinking: have you been reviewing past resentments? Reliving negative experiences?
- Come to the present moment.
- Focus on the positive. What is good right now?
- Who are you reaching for? Think about the kind of person you want to become. What would that person do right now?
- Interview the craving. "Who are you, and what do you want here?" Is it hunger, thirst, stress, the presence of your trigger foods, or an uncomfortable feeling? What do you really need?

- Ask the wise recovering person inside you to tell you what would help. Or ask yourself what a sponsor or mentor would say—or call one and ask.

- Make a box—a pretty one that fits in the area of your home where your cravings usually strike. Fill the box with hints, reminders, and things you can do to distract yourself from the craving. You might consider a journal, tablet, or note pad and pen; a mandala coloring book and crayons, or crossword puzzles; Sudoku, a Rubik's cube; small puzzles, a small container of putty; a prayer . . . the Prayer of St. Francis, the Third or Seventh Step; friends; a game on your phone—anything that works for you. Then, when you have a craving, open the box and enjoy!

When you are having a craving, remind yourself, "This is time limited. I will not be feeling this craving forever. It's worth it to me to not give in because it will enable me to get everything I really want."

Trigger Situations

Now, let's talk about the situations that set off your inappropriate eating in response to your addiction. First is loneliness. I have yet to meet a food addict who isn't lonely. They may not call loneliness a hole in their soul, but I would claim otherwise. Some food addicts use isolation and loneliness more than others; all those with addictive disorders seem to have a kind of emptiness that hurts, and they try to fill the emptiness with food and other things. If you're self-isolating, you are triggering yourself.

Existential malaise aside, there are some trigger situations will always drive you to create cravings and discomfort—the call from your mother-in-law or from your boss, for example.

Triggers will happen. If you ignore them long enough, they will grow into cravings. Note, if you will, these situations are not often solved by food.

> **Triggers will happen. If you ignore them long enough, they will grow into cravings.**

You first need to recognize the trigger when it happens. You may experience an unsettled feeling in your belly, or a situation that plays on loop in your mind, or that all too familiar sense that you're dealing with someone who simply does not understand.

The more triggers you experience, the more susceptible you are to cravings and relapse. That's why I have a rule: one trigger means, "Oops! I need to talk with someone about it now." Two triggers mean you need to talk about it *and* pray about it. Three triggers mean you need to talk about it, pray about it, consult a trusted advocate, decide how to act, then act.

There are lots of ways to act when you are confronting a trigger situation. Let's say you have to visit that relative, who invariably triggers you and puts you at risk for a relapse. Set up someone to talk to after you leave.

If there is a buffet of your drug foods, perhaps call a friend from the ladies' room; ask your Higher Power for help; go sit in another room and talk with dear Aunt Tillie.

If your hostess burns chocolate chip cookie dough candles while you're there, that's a triple whammy. Perhaps you pray; perhaps you find a way to unobtrusively blow it out; perhaps you go hug Aunt Tillie, make your exit, then make that phone call on the way home.

> **EXERCISE: Identify your most common triggers**

Sit down, right here and right now, and make a list: at least a dozen of your most common triggers, and at least a dozen actions you can take to resolve them.

If you're looking for action ideas, borrow from one of my clients:

- One recovering client told me she sat on her kitchen floor and asked her Higher Power to come get her; she waited; her Higher Power came.
- Another said, "I called my sponsor; she said she'd be right over. And she came with another friend and saved me."
- Another said, "I got in the bathtub and stayed there a long time, crying, till it passed."

You Are in Recovery

A craving is a powerful urge to do the thing you do not want to do. A trigger is a less powerful warning that it's coming. Both triggers and cravings can be physical, mental, emotional, or spiritual in origin. But believe me, they are very, very real. Which is why you need a regular recovery program. You must consistently evaluate your eating plan and your behavior. And a big part of your success depends on how you choose to view your addiction and refusing to go it alone.

I was speaking with a man who was forty-two years sober, and he said this, "I think being an addict is the most precious gift of all; we who are addicts have a hole inside us that only God can fill; we became addicts by trying to fill that hole with sugar, flour, fat, salt, alcohol, drugs, whatever." He likes to think about the idea that God put that hole in us because God wanted to be with us and in us. And that hole, that emptiness, that loneliness, that hunger for God is a precious gift. "It carved out my soul enough that God could fit inside."

If you think about food addiction this way, rather than thinking about it as an emptiness—resenting that emptiness, being defiant about that emptiness, trying to fill that emptiness with food and other drugs—you'll find it easier to let a Higher Power in.

> **EXERCISE: Take regular stock of your program**

Answer the following questions, particularly when you are experiencing frequent cravings or encountering triggers.

- Are you eating some foods that aren't quite good enough for you?
- Are you allowing yourself to obsess or ruminate?
- Are you speaking rudely to yourself, blaming yourself, putting yourself down?
- Are there feelings you need to process or handle?
- Do you let yourself cry or feel and express your feelings in other ways?
- Do you have people you trust to talk things out with?
- Are you working on a spiritual program?
- Have you tried meditation, reading and writing, fellowship?
- Do you have enough emotional and spiritual support?

Make another list: what do you need to do to protect yourself or rescue yourself?

And one more: what are your challenges to the transformation you're seeking?

You must talk with others you trust about your triggers and cravings. This is hard work. It is never perfect and not always in your control. But you can learn to manage it and live a life of joy and freedom.

When Slips Become a Struggle

This means your response to your last slip was inadequate.
You must do MORE or do DIFFERENTLY
in order to avoid progression to full relapse.
It also means, by definition, you need the help of other people to reestablish
stable abstinence.
TO NOT ALLOW OTHERS TO HELP YOU AT THIS STAGE IS TO BUY A TICKET ON THE RELAPSE EXPRESS!
The question is – how to tell what to do.
It takes thought, decision, action to put down the food at this stage.
Your ability to tolerate the drug foods increases, and your mind gradually loses the ability to think and reason clearly about anything.

Chapter 8

Boundaries

Once upon a time there was a caterpillar who ate and ate until he was greatly obese (or so he'd be if he were human). He curled up in his chrysalis, the quiet place he created, and inside, transformed himself from a stout little caterpillar into a colorful flying butterfly. That process of transformation is what you're beginning here. You are establishing a new, healthy lifestyle. You're in recovery from food addiction, so you'll need to create and continue daily practices to support your reclaimed health and set wise boundaries and clear guidelines with yourself, food, and other people. You will need to set up new patterns of attitudes and behaviors that will help you maintain your new lifestyle so you can become who you are meant to grow into. And that means setting boundaries.

A boundary, if you recall, is a limit set between you and another person, object, or situation. A boundary is an invisible line between your choices, needs, and responsibilities and those of others.

Abusive eating makes boundaries unclear, so if you get confused

> Abusive eating makes boundaries unclear, so if you get confused during the recovery process, there's a good reason.

during the recovery process, there's a good reason. There are all the food boundaries you were taught in childhood; there are the dozens of diets you may have tried and abusive food behaviors you accumulated; there are all sorts of emotional boundaries with food and other people, both in and out of abstinence and recovery. You may use food and eating behaviors instead of maintaining personal boundaries, and it keeps you from learning to effectively maintain personal boundaries. It prevents you from learning new ways to care for yourself. It keeps you from learning how to comfortably maintain your new boundaries. And it keeps others confused or unsure and makes it seem okay for them to violate your new boundaries. Messy, to be sure.

Creating boundaries will bring up unpleasant feelings. You may have a hard time rearranging your life to allow for proper foods. This will be a learning experience. It will take time, and you may make mistakes. Setting effective boundaries—with yourself, the food, and others—and stating them clearly, with limits and consequences, will allow you to become who you are meant to be. As with anything in life, the longer you persist at setting boundaries, the easier it will get.

The Boundary Between You and Food

Since food molecules become the molecules of your heart, lungs, liver, brain, and other organs, changing your relationship with food is one of the most important things you can do. You need to do it with care and respect for the body. One way you go about that is by setting boundaries.

> **Food boundaries protect you from binges, purges, and a whole lot of uncomfortable feelings and conditions (not to mention, weight gain).**

I've said it before, and I'll say it again: food boundaries protect you from binges, purges, and a whole lot of uncomfortable feelings and conditions (not to mention, weight gain). Food boundaries keep you from negative energies, help you learn to value yourself, and give you the freedom to learn to become comfortable in your own skin.

==Your food boundaries are yours on a very personal level==. It takes time, thought, and work to learn how to protect yourself. Truly, some foods cost a lot and hurt you. You must say no, mean no, and maintain that no. Even if society and others around you offer this or that—thinking it's good or fun or helpful—still say, "No." You don't want to upset, hurt, or offend other people, and you don't want to cause or receive negative feelings. But the first boundary you draw is inside yourself. It's a blunt refusal to allow the body, mind, and spirit to be harmed using inappropriate foods. If it seems as though I'm repeating myself, it's because I am—it's that important.

As touched upon in Chapter 6, boundaries can be of different strengths, which are even more nuanced than our pendulum swing:

- There is the red barbed wire boundary: "Nuh-uh, no way am I doing *that*."
- The real red boundary: "No honey, not in a million years." No barbed wire, just serious intent and determination.
- The orange: "Boy, I could get in big trouble here."
- The yellow: "Better not cross that."
- The green: "Yeah, this is safe."
- The lush, deep green: "Oh, are we going to love this."

Barbed wire boundaries with yourself and with food are especially important because they affect your ability to establish healthy boundaries elsewhere in your life.

Boundaries are not necessarily permanent. You are allowed to change them if they are not working for you or if a unique situation requires it. That does not mean you shift in a way that allows using your binge or drug foods again; it means you learn to make changes to accommodate the situation in which you find yourself and still maintain your food boundaries.

Boundaries with Yourself

What makes you who you are? What do you need from your food, your life, and other people to handle and reach your food goals? Knowing the answers to these questions is essential for your transformation.

The boundaries you set for yourself need to be ones with which you are most comfortable. Some boundaries are only in your mind: focusing on your core beliefs, letting go of false beliefs, changing what you think of yourself and others. This is why I devoted an entire chapter (Chapter 2: Start with How You Think) to your mindset. These boundaries need to be clear, practiced regularly, and familiar; you need to experience their value. You must be completely committed to maintaining your boundaries with yourself. You allow your spirit to heal by being congruent. You experience peace when your behavior is consistent with your words, body language, or intentions.

Boundaries protect your life and preserve your highest potential, which allows your ultimate purpose to be fulfilled. So, regardless of the curveballs that come your way (and they will), keep in mind:

- Abusive eating is using food or food products in a way that is harmful to the body, mind, and spirit or self. This includes compulsive eating, dieting, bingeing, purging, starving, eating to manage feelings, eating for punishment, etc.

- Abstinent eating is all about following the principles of the food plan and moving toward deeper recovery. This is a careful process of hard work, change, and growth. It is rarely perfect. You make mistakes, learn lessons from them, and move on.

> **There is a lesson to be learned from every mistake.**

Did you catch that? There is a lesson to be learned from every mistake. If you mess up, slip, or stumble, go back in your mind to what happened before the mistake and figure out what caused it and what you need to change.

EXERCISE: Set your initial boundaries

1. What are your abstinence boundaries? In other words, what rules must you follow in order to maintain your abstinence (i.e., if you break them, you will no longer be abstinent)?

    Is this boundary firm, flexible, or movable?

2. What are the principles of your recovery program to which you know you need to adhere to stay abstinent?

    Is this boundary firm, flexible, or movable?

Sometimes you create boundaries with yourself that hurt; they hurt your feelings or make you feel deprived and unhappy. "I can't live without this food," some of my clients will say. Sometimes, when the positivity fades away, the conversations in your mind become painful.

- I hate my body weight. I don't want to give up all the foods I love just to weigh a normal weight.
- This abstinence idea seems more like deprivation than healing.
- I don't want to spend the rest of my life without sugar.

Such thoughts indicate something is missing. You have not found a solution that will work for the problem. You need to broaden the search for the positive and maybe adjust your boundaries. Until you find a food plan that really works for you, allowing your boundaries to be a bit more flexible (less specific) may help.

To do so, look at what you really want and point your thoughts in that general direction:

- I choose to eat food that nourishes my body and keeps me healthy.
- I want my cravings and obsessions to stop.
- I choose to eat with dignity and self-respect—to sit down, taste the food, and enjoy it.
- Eating in a healthier way is good for my body, mind, and spirit.
- This is so hard, and it hurts so bad, that I'm struggling to stay level and calm, and that's okay too.
- My body is a gift, given to help me create a life of joy, growth, and service. I want to treat my body with respect and care.

Once you have adopted a food plan that works for you, you can create more specific boundaries.

Relationship Boundaries

Let's pretend you have been struggling with your weight for most of your life. And let's pretend you have tried many of the weight loss programs out there; you've lost weight lots of times, only to (sadly) regain it. (Hopefully now, finally, you've moved beyond trying to solve the symptom to believe in, accept, and deal with the real problem.)

What do you think others in your life think and feel about your situation: will they accuse you of experimenting with a new, creative way to say "starvation and self-abuse" when you talk about abstinence? (If that doesn't shake your commitment and resolve and make you question the whole addiction thing, nothing will.) Will they think you haven't enough willpower? Are they inconvenienced by being asked to provide you with special foods when you are following a plan? In the past, were they frustrated watching you overeat when not following a plan; did they wonder why you had to have more when eating a single serving was so easy for them?

Of all our experiences, relationships with other people can be the most comfortable and most deeply rewarding. They can also be the most difficult, time-consuming, desperate struggles of our lives. Especially around food, eating, and body weight.

In recovery, other people's reactions to your food choices can become an issue. Change is threatening to everyone sometimes, particularly your abstinence from insane foods and behaviors. You'll need to accept that. Others may be curious, annoyed, or upset by the food changes you're making. Dealing with others about your food, eating, and body weight can be difficult, painful, and embarrassing. No one wants to hear, "Okay, here we go again, back on another crazy diet." No one wants to face, "Can't you have just one? I made them special for you." Even the nasty voice in your head (some call it ego, or addiction, or monkey mind) can join in with insults. I am often deeply moved by the client's feelings about food and their fear of other people's opinions surrounding their choices and boundaries. "What will they think of me?!"

First of all, "abstinent" boundaries tend to impact others. They may be asked to accommodate your changes, need to change their own behavior, or are faced with behaviors they should change. They may be unable to believe the restrictions are necessary or appropriate; they may legitimately worry about your health and safety.

If you change the boundaries you have with food irregularly and/or without warning, it may upset others who are planning to prepare food or eat a meal with you. But the fact is, sometimes you need to change the boundaries; sometimes you need to set aside what you have been doing. And sometimes you need to experiment with different ways of eating until you find what really works for you. This can be confusing for the people who love you; it's important you let them know when you make changes. The goal is to be able to enjoy being together and caring for each other.

Boundaries are never an excuse to be selfish, impossible, or arrogant; you never refuse to help someone in real need, but they are a choice, just as the food plan is a choice and relating to others effectively is a choice. You need to know what your boundaries are, and you need to have thought about how best to discuss the boundaries with others. That means knowing how to enforce your boundaries with yourself first, not obsessing about other people's feelings, and how you do not want to hurt them.

Not All Relationships are Created Equal

The way we handle people and their responses to our food, eating, and body weight should be different based on our relationships with them. There are different levels of relationships, and that means different levels of boundaries.

Many years ago, Anne Katherine, author of *Where to Draw the Line: How to Set Healthy Boundaries Every Day*, divided boundaries into four areas: Acquaintance, Neighbor, Comrade, Intimate. She claimed that we need to change our responses and our behavior around these different types in any given situation. The degree and depth of your relationship, she said, define its context, and what you share with someone close to you ought to be very much dependent on how close they are to you.[1]

What you tell someone who has known and loved you for a long time is different from what you tell someone you barely know. Consider the context of the relationship. You don't regale your boss with a story of the argument you had with your mother-in-law. It won't help your career. And your dentist is not likely to be able to help with your tax problems. Choose to discuss what is in the normal scope of your relationship; try to keep the relationship where it belongs in your feelings about the person without allowing yourself to be criticized or walked over.

What to Say When Asked

So, what do you say when someone offers a suggestion, asks a question, or comments on your food plan? First, think about your rela-

---

[1.] Anne Katherine, Where to Draw the Line (Fireside, original ed. edition, 2000).

tionship with the person to whom you're speaking. If the person is a coworker, an acquaintance, not someone you care about or rely on, your response may be as simple as, "Thanks for sharing; yes, I'm at it again; what do you do for fun in your life?"

If the person is an employer, or someone you value but don't know well, a simple, "Yes, that's true," might handle the question. If they ask what program you're following, you might say, "I'm working with this really weird/really brilliant dietitian (or doctor or program) who says I have allergies to lots of foods and I need to be really careful till we sort it all out." Answer questions, but don't rehash. Tell the truth, but you are not required to give the *whole* truth.

Be patient; trust is created by actions, not words. Change takes time for everyone. Allow a bit of space to accept the changes you are now making. If needed, provide reassurance about your commitment to the relationship. Be consistent and patient, allowing the other person time and space for feelings.

A caution here: in several situations, those asking me such questions were in desperate need; they were looking for help with their own food problems. Don't miss a cry for help. Try saying something like, "Why do you ask? Are you concerned about something?"

Then there are family members and others who have watched you struggle and suffer for years. Some of them may be very supportive; some may enjoy teasing or throwing out critical comments. There is no one way to handle these, but you need to do it with dignity and self-respect. Sometimes a blank stare may work, sometimes a quiet word. Sometimes you may need to leave the room.

Then we come to the folk that Anne Katherine, author of *Boundaries: Where You End and I Begin,* calls Intimates.[2] These are

---

[2] Anne Katherine, *Boundaries: Where You End and I Begin—How to Recognize and Set Healthy Boundaries* (Hazelden Publishing, 1994).

the people you trust with your thoughts and feelings. You should have two to four (maybe more) people in your life with whom you feel safe to talk about your feelings—your hurts, joys, goals. They are the ones you trust not to reveal to others things that might be used to hurt you. They really listen and help you move toward your goals. They may teach, coach, support, and validate you. They may have special skills to help when you need it. Hold these people close to you. They are the precious ones. Hold them close and be grateful for their presence.

Codependence

But let's get to a core issue many face: it's called codependence. Perhaps you've heard of it. You may know it as an unhealthy attachment to another person. Regarding your boundaries, this is a term that describes a relationship where you allow someone else to push your buttons.

In the book, *Waking Up Just in Time*, Rabbi Abraham J. Twerski, M.D., says, "Rather than determining your own course in life, you react to another person's behavior, essentially allowing that person to manipulate your actions . . . it can occur in any situation where you surrender your own thinking and your own decision-making to someone else."[3]

No one can protect you from the consequences of your eating behavior. You have choices of what foods you eat, but once you eat them, you have no control over what they do in your body. So, when you change your behavior to please others and hurt yourself in the process, that's codependence. You have the right to choose your own

---

[3] Abraham J. Twerski, Waking Up Just in Time: A Therapist Shows How to Use the Twelve Steps Approach to Life's Ups and Downs (St. Martin's Griffin, 1995).

feelings and behavior, and you are allowed to eat the foods your body needs.

> **Obesity is the symptom, the cause, or the result of some other problem.**

You need to remind yourself that sixty-five percent of America is overweight and obese. Obesity is the symptom, the cause, or the result of some other problem. Dealing with your food issues, whatever they are, is the best way to lead yourself to a state of health and well-being . . . as well as a normal body weight. People who do not have issues with food and eating usually don't have issues with what you eat.

Taking care of yourself and your body is the most important thing you need to do. Being whole is what enables you to be available for the relationships and growth you want and need.

So, set yourself up for success. Call back your power.

Refuse to put yourself in a submissive, harassed, or abused state of mind. Change the words you say to yourself and others about food. You may be tempted to say, "I'm not allowed; I need to give up . . ." Instead, turn it toward the positive: "I realized I am allergic to _____; I no longer eat _____; I decided to stay off _____ for a while; I decided to kick _____ out of my food plan; no, not today, thank you." Now you are in control. This is your choice, and you have the power.

All-Purpose Answers to "Have Some of this Food"

You have the right to refuse to eat food you do not want to put in your body. And here are a few examples of what, exactly, you can say when someone asks you to do otherwise (and "have some of this food"):

No, thank you.
I'm not eating _____ this month.
No, thank you.
I know you worked really hard to make it just for me, and I'm sure it's excellent, but I'm not ready to eat it right now.
No, thank you.
I gave it up for (Lent/Passover last month), and it felt so good I decided to keep going.
No, thank you.
I'm working with this really weird nutritionist, and she wants me to stay off _____ for right now.
No, thank you.
And the way I've lost it is by not eating _____.
No, thank you.
I love you dearly; you're my favorite (aunt, uncle, cousin?) but I'm not going to eat that now.
No, thank you.
It was delicious, but I'm full.
No, thank you.
I've had enough.
No, thank you.
You're putting that on the wrong plate; I'm not eating it.
No, thank you.
Why is it so important to you that I eat this?
No, thank you.
What part of "No, thank you" did you not understand?
My crazy nutritionist says if I can get people like you to call and talk to her about your problems with my food plan, she'll give me a free session. Would you do that for me? It will save me a lot of money!

Smoothing the Way with Family

I believe up to eighty percent of the problems with drawing food boundaries today are rooted in your food experiences as a child. The first step is figuring out what they were and why they were put there; the second step is coming to peace with what you are choosing to do today.

Your family taught you a lot about boundaries, including those with food and eating. Did you eat at the kitchen table, in front of the TV, in the car? When you ate in public, did you need to sit down or were you allowed to walk with the food while eating? Were your meals regular? Did you need to clean your plate, finish your vegetables? Was Sunday dinner special? What about on vacation or at the beach? What other social or emotional issues have changed your eating patterns?

In one way or another, each of these sets a boundary around food. Good, bad, or otherwise, you need to consider whether they hamper or support your current goals and how to make changes, if needed.

> **EXERCISE: Evaluate your old boundaries**

Old boundaries are going to pop up again throughout your recovery process, so it pays to know what they are, then plan for them. Here's a way for you to evaluate:

- List some food boundaries you learned in childhood that are helpful or not helpful to you now.
- What was the code? What was not okay? What was your belief around food and eating?

- What influence did relatives, teachers, and other adults have on these family rules?
- What influence did your peers have?
- How have years of dieting and weight regain affected your food boundaries?

We want to teach our children to treasure themselves, but sometimes it doesn't work out that way. Children are taught to set up lines around their lives in the way that seems best. If you were treated as willful or disobedient when you expressed a contrary opinion, you may have built up walls, not boundaries, and others may struggle to relate to you.

In addition, family members tend to follow a script, and what they say or how they behave is based on the roles they play. Anything that upsets that script may cause hurt or division—at the very least, it can make for an awkward situation. And that's hard. If you don't know what to do about it, you may revert to the tried and familiar, which you likely do not want to do.

Here are a few suggestions for when you're about to enter a difficult situation (namely, when you're about to break the rules you grew up with, particularly among close family and friends):

- Be honest, but do not make a big production of your meal.
- Plan ahead. Be certain the food you can eat will be available.
- Be prepared to remove yourself if you need to.
- Eat a snack—before you go—in case the meal is delayed.
- When someone asks you an awkward question, ask a question in return: "Why do you ask?"

- Tell the truth, but you do not need to say the whole truth.
- Understand that others may feel threatened by your food changes (especially if they know they should be doing the same).
- Make a joke: "I'm following this weird allergy dietitian I found on the internet; it's strange, but it is helping my itchy skin (or headaches or anger level) a lot."

EXERCISE: Recognize boundary violations

Think back to a time when someone close to you made it difficult to follow your food plan, made it seem like your choices were an imposition. It can help you prepare for future incidents. The following will get you started:

- Write a short summary of a food boundary violation situation.
- List four possible motivations for the violator.
- What is your goal in this situation?
- Create some possible responses for each of the motivations.

Moving On

Now that you're an adult, you get to draw a line around your food and your life because it is *your* life. You get to draw boundaries around your food behavior because this affects your life. You get to choose how you live and grow and develop. You get to make choices for your one and only life.

At times, you may choose to tighten your boundaries for a while if you are doing difficult emotional work, coming out of a bad emotional space, needing to focus on your step work. At these times, you may want to be extra vigilant about your usual meals and snacks. You may want to be more careful about timing, quality, and content of meals. You may want to increase other aspects of your recovery program as well.

The key is to avoid making your regular food plan boundaries so tight and rigid that you cannot live your life in freedom and comfort. If you feel imprisoned, you will fight to be released. If you feel limited and restricted, it will bring back the "diet trauma" and keep you from getting free.

> **The key is to avoid making your regular food plan boundaries so tight and rigid that you cannot live your life in freedom and comfort.**

Above all, you want to protect the ideas you value and create a life you're happy with.

Setting boundaries (and sticking to them) may be irksome at times. It may require you to call out for a meal, bring your meal with you, plan your food ahead of time, or respectfully decline a food that harms you. Be prepared. Come up with a few "explanations" that work for you. They could be straight forward: "I just want to eat more nutritious food; I'm finding that sugared and processed food does not make me feel well." They may keep with your sense of humor: "Why yes, I am starting a new exercise program—you may not recognize me the next time you see me!" And remember, no boundary needs to be permanent unless you want it that way. Choose your boundaries for yourself and your recovery, your well-being and your spiritual growth and freedom.

It's Up to You

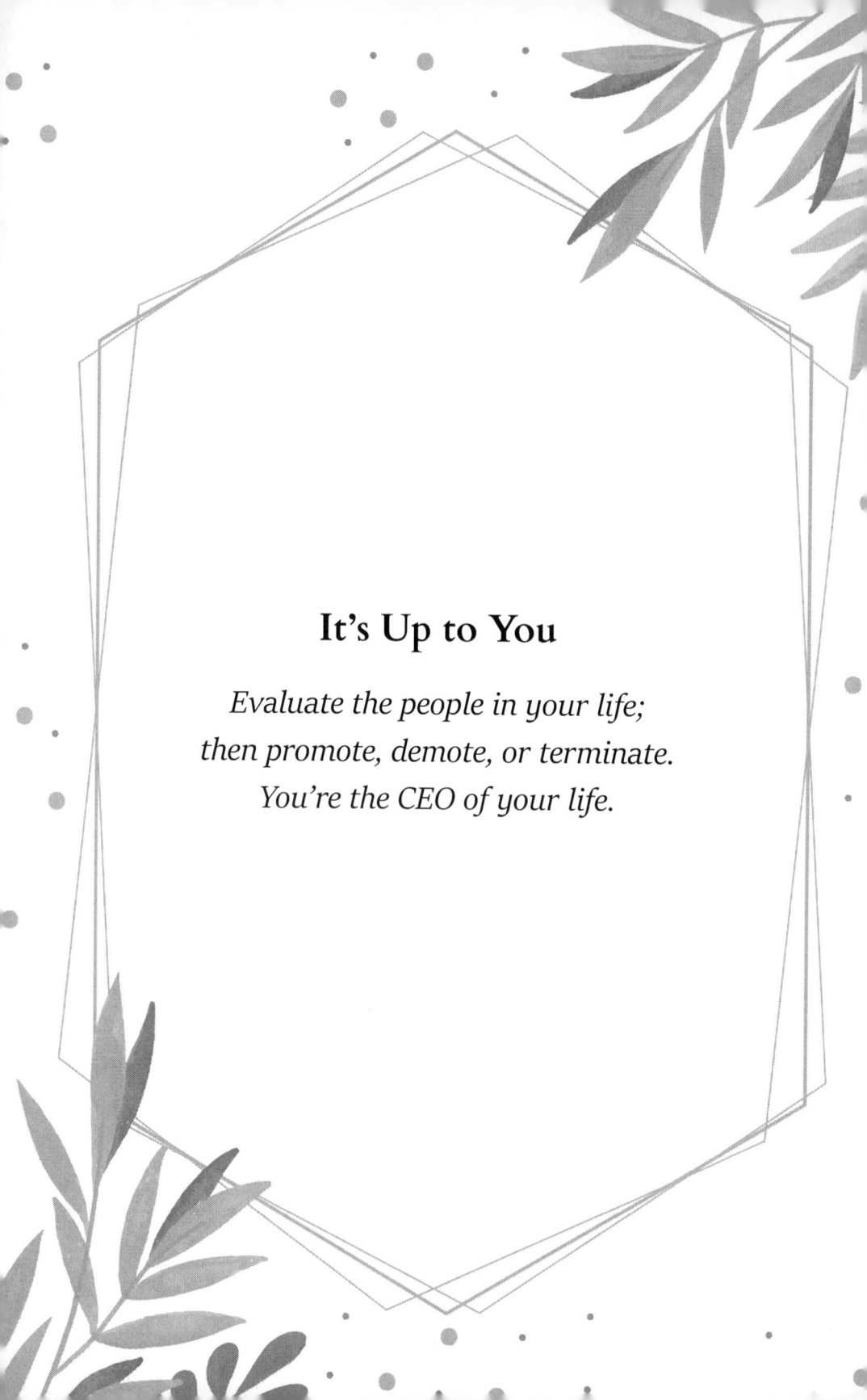

*Evaluate the people in your life;
then promote, demote, or terminate.
You're the CEO of your life.*

Chapter 9
Daily Practices

Following your new food plan may be hard at first. Let me reassure you: any time you want to make a major change in your life, it's hard, and it hurts. That's part of being human. You followed your other behaviors because they worked in some way; they provided some benefit. For example, food may have pushed down or shut off hurtful feelings. You now know this is not solving the problem; the feeling is still there and will come up to hurt you again and again. Just "not eating" when the painful feeling comes up, however, is very painful and difficult. Thankfully, you are willing to change because those behaviors do not work in a way that is helpful to you.

In real life, it's easier to create a new behavior than to resist and abstain from an old one. A habit is hard to break. On the other hand, it takes focus and effort to establish a new behavior, but it can be done—not by fighting or resisting your usual habits, but by setting

> **It takes focus and effort to establish a new behavior, but it can be done—not by fighting or resisting your usual habits, but by setting up a whole new system of behavior that will keep you from needing to eat abusively.**

up a whole new system of behavior that will keep you from needing to eat abusively. That is your daily practice.

People do a lot of different things to maintain their abstinence and equilibrium in the long-term, and they regularly change what they're doing to fit the needs of the day or week. It also depends on their personal goals, what they want to achieve in the subsequent weeks or months, what they value, and what their stressors are. But most everyone has a consistent set of practices that they indulge in each day.

First, you need to know the basic principles of food recovery so you can better understand the holistic daily practices ahead.

Principles of Food Recovery

Self-Care. Do the things that need to be done to take care of you. When you're eating abusively, what do you neglect: your nails, hair, house, hobbies, other commitments—your joy? Focus on what's important; focus on taking care of you.

Structure. Set up your life so that it's possible to be or to become the person you want to be. To do so, you must plan time to care for the body, mind, and spirit. This includes rest and comforting activities. Rest means enough sleep, but also it means emotional and spiritual rest, allowing yourself time for what you need, for what gives you comfort and joy. And time to exercise the body so it can remain strong and effective for you.

Support. Find people who can meet your emotional needs and support you in your struggles. Addicts are all isolators. So, you need to learn to identify and create supportive relationships that work for you. You need folks you can trust enough to tell difficult truths to and know they won't be used to harm you. You may need effective professional support as well; you may need to find advisers, coaches, and advocates—people who can care for you effectively. (Check out the chapter on trusted advisers, Chapter 10: Support Network.)

Spirituality. Find and know how to access a force outside of yourself willing to help. Not to be confused with a religious program; it might be a Higher Power, God, Yahweh, or the Universe. Read, meditate, pray to stay focused in the right direction. And learn to listen to your intuition, your "Inner Core of Wisdom," or the "Wise Person Within." Take some time each day to sit quietly—pray, meditate, or get in touch with the power within you or the person you want to become.

The Sane Food Plan. Find a food plan that really works for you, one that meets your nutrient, hunger, and energy needs, corrects any food-related illnesses, and leads you to your healthy body weight.

Sustainability. Make sure your food goals are sustainable, meaning your food plan will work for you long-term and can be adjusted when needed. It's something you can be comfortable following every day. And it's integrated, allowing you to meet the rest of your goals to create the joyful, useful life that you've always dreamt about.

Dr. Marty Lerner, PhD, started a rehab in Florida many years ago. He has an acronym for these behaviors that I like a lot: SMERF. It stands for the following:

S stands for Spirituality. It's a word with a lot of meanings. For here and now, please think about the ageless, timeless, eternal "you" or the "Wise Person Within"—the person you really are and want to become. Religion, yes, if it works for you. Any spiritual program that puts you in touch with who you are and who you want to become. This includes some daily time to consider your needs and values, to be in tune with yourself, to meditate or pray, or simply think your own thoughts.

S also stands for Self Care. We often put the needs of everyone else ahead of our own, and we don't let ourselves have the time or space to do what will help us: getting a haircut or pedicure, taking the time to chat with a friend, taking a nap, buying that special item we have wanted, being well enough and clear headed enough to do a good job at work, asking someone to do what they should have done already, asking for help when you need it, taking a break when you need it . . . well, you get the idea. The key is to take care of you.

M is for Meetings. This is a general term; it means a group of people who understand you, who you trust, who have things in common with you, who believe in you, who support your goals. There is a whole chapter in this book about creating trusted advisers and using a variety of support groups (Chapter 10: Support Network). Keep searching and interviewing till you find a variety of people who relate well to you and are able to meet your needs.

E is for Exercise. You may not sit quietly in front of the TV, computer, and other electronic objects all day. Burning calories happens most rapidly in the muscles. Use them or lose them; the body won't maintain what's not often used. So, find a way to get some movement in each day, even if it means you walk around the rooms of your house, put dishes in the dishwasher, or do an online yoga, exercise, or belly dancing class. (Do you realize how good belly dancing is for flexibility, stretching, and fun? It burns calories too!) Or volunteer with Habitat for Humanity or another charity—and help your body, as well as those in need within your community.

R is for Rest. Take care of all the things important to your body. Get enough sleep, but also have enough time to enjoy whatever allows you to kick back and relax. It may be reading, traveling, knitting, or being with friends.

F is the Food Plan. We have discussed this at length. Find one that meets your requirements and follow it. Take out all your binge and drug foods and their cousins and friends. If you make a mistake, get back on plan at the next meal or snack—then take a deep breath and look back. What caused that problem; what were you feeling, wanting, looking for; what can you do to avoid it next time? What food plan would be best for you? This is your choice. Many are available. *Your Personal Food Plan Guide* contains a number of different food plans, lists of the different foods in each category, and suggestions for choosing or creating one that works for you. You'll find information on this at the back of this book.

And what do you really want to accomplish in your life? For me, it was this book. That meant I had to allocate the time to sit down regularly and write—or research, or review, or edit. This must be put in the plan, too.

Daily Recovery Practices

Food addiction is a physical, biochemical illness you're contending with. It doesn't go away. Dealing with this kind of food addiction/food sensitivity means you need to create a practice of daily living that is different from what and how you do your life today—one that sends the obsession with food out every available door and window.

> **Food addiction is a physical, biochemical illness you're contending with. It doesn't go away.**

Your goal is to manage your recovery in a way that enhances your life, lets you create the life you really want, and fits well into your daily routine. It's not perfect, it never will be, and it needs to change with your work, family situation, and your own needs.

The purpose of a daily recovery practice is to provide a new structure for your day. In a nutshell, you replace your food obsession with healthy activities. As you'll see, this includes developing a relationship with your Higher Power. Why? Because putting down the food can let in some nasty feelings; you'll need to deal with those. If you need a new life, your Higher Power accepts trade-ins, any condition.

> **In a nutshell, you replace your food obsession with healthy activities.**

Here's a list of activities with which to structure your daily recovery practice, and the time of day you might indulge yourself with them:

Mostly in the morning

- Read a meditation book
- Write a response to the reading
- Recite the steps you're studying today
- Breathe in the Spirit
- Write a gratitude list
- Write a third step list—a list of all those things you cannot fix
- Speak with a sponsor, friend, or trusted advisor
- Read a text of your religion (the Bible, the Torah, the Koran)

Throughout the day

- Read Twelve Step literature
- Pray
- Meditate
- Journal
- Breathe deeply and spiritually
- Put God in the passenger seat and simply chat
- Write a mantra
- Color a mandala
- Exercise; focus your mind on a meditation
- Sing a song
- Speak with a trusted advisor
- Make a team of five strong friends
- Plan healthy appropriate foods
- Evaluate your schedule; adjust it so it's workable
- Ask your Higher Power's opinion about a decision
- Put a reminder of you Higher Power on your desk; touch base with your Higher Power when you see it—put a short reminder in your schedule book, or schedule an alarm
- Sign up for a daily meditation by email
- Write a reply to the meditation
- Give and get hugs appropriately
- Allow time to get to your appointments without rushing
- Create twenty minutes to sit in the sunshine
- Plan time to eat meals leisurely

- Chat with a friend
- Invite your Higher Power for a cup of tea
- Indulge in your favorite hobby
- Go to a support group or a Twelve Step Meeting
- Schedule a half hour rest period in your day

Mostly in the evening

- Evaluate the day: what part of it went beautifully; what made it go well? What part fell apart; what would work better next time?
- What patterns do you see in the day?
- Can you find your Higher Power's fingerprints in the day?
- Write a short gratitude list
- Write a list of things you would like your Higher Power to take care of while you sleep
- Read something nourishing
- Hug yourself or give yourself some comfort
- Breathe, breathe, breathe
- Create a ritual that pleases you
- Go to sleep early enough to wake refreshed and rested

Now that you have an idea about what to do, the question is how to get it into your daily life in an effective way. Activities need to fit into your daily plan somehow. Start with a calendar numbered by hours. Put in your mealtimes. Give yourself time of prayer, quiet, reflection, or self-soothing each day if that's a new behavior for you.

Find the time to purchase and prepare your appropriate foods. (Don't panic, there's a whole chapter on that.) Plan eating times; if you feel you have no set times to eat, you need to ask whether this is a way that your abusive food behavior is supported and how to change that. Focus: set up your daily schedule to allow time for the changes you want to make in your life to fit comfortably. You want enough time for the healthy behaviors while keeping yourself joyfully occupied in your vulnerable times.

Think it through. For example, consider your food plan when you're fitting in your workout time—you want to have enough energy to exercise but not be overfull or over hungry.

Add anything else you want to your daily practice and pay attention to the timing. If it's too tight, it may feel like an oppressive ball of chores. Relax, you can change it any time. Once a week, take time to look at your schedule and see what is working and what isn't. Make the changes needed. Your daily practice should feel like a supportive guidebook.

Every Day is Different

Give yourself the freedom to change your daily practice any time you feel the need. Look at your goals right now; try to find activities that help you get the relationship you want.

Remember that your spiritual practice is likely to be diminished before your food is negatively affected. Learn to use these behaviors to protect your food abstinence and recovery.

Creating a daily recovery practice is part of establishing a spiritual lifestyle, which is what will lead you to freedom from food obsession. Remember that recovery is a journey, not a destination, and be prepared to be flexible and innovative in your activities.

There will also be spells where a different level of recovery practice is required.

Many people define three levels of their recovery practice . . .

Basic, or Bottom Line: the minimum amount needed to stay comfortably abstinent. When chaos abounds, what do you really need? Keep to this area for no longer than a week. By two weeks, you may need intensive care.

Normal: your usual, comfortable space. It's where you feel good, and your world is moving along well.

Intensive Care: problems or stresses are surfacing. You need to increase support and self-care.

Normal Recovery Practices

A normal recovery practice for many involves taking time in the morning to meditate or pray; you might journal, read a specific book, or workout. Most of the workday starts a bit later in the morning, then lunch, maybe a workout—a walk, a trip to the gym. Support groups may meet at this time, as well. Most people benefit from creating a group of people who know them well, care about them, support them, understand the disease, and are available to listen and help or guide them. Lastly, take time for the things you enjoy—family, friends, alone time. Rest. Get a good night's sleep.

Intensive Care

When things start going wrong—you're struggling with everyday life; feelings are coming up and you need time to process them; you see a relapse coming down the track; you're just recovering from a slip, jump, or relapse—put yourself in intensive care.

What does that mean? Well, for most addicts, self-care is the hardest thing they do. They sacrifice their own needs to the demands of others or to their own beliefs about the wishes of others (true or not). In doing so, they give up their right to the things they really need for their survival and well-being.

I'm guessing the same holds true for you:

- You suffer.
- You feel pain.
- You need comfort.
- You relapse to stop the pain.
- Then you have two problems.
- And the pain is twice as big.

When you see this cycle beginning, take a time out: take time off from work; cancel any non-urgent commitments. (If it does not involve a trip to the emergency room, death, dismemberment, or the IRS, it's not urgent.) Take time for yourself for seven to fourteen days. Give yourself the opportunity to rest and renew.

What does this include? It can be anything (or many things) of your choice. Here are a few suggestions:

- Seven support meetings in seven days
- A daily nap
- Eight hours of sleep per night
- Half an hour of prayer and meditation daily
- Manicure, pedicure, haircut, facial, massage

- Lunch with a supportive friend
- Daily exercise
- Step work
- Let the sun warm your heart
- Journal daily
- Walk in the moonlight
- Weigh and measure all your food
- A gratitude list
- A list titled, "Your Job, God"
- Half an hour to do whatever you want
- A daily indulgence
- A new recovery manual, book, or workbook

During this time, make the opportunity to talk with people you trust about what's going on with you; listen to their advice and consider it. At the end of this time, make time to reassess your situation with a trusted adviser and decide how to proceed in a way that enhances your recovery. Trust me, I am part of these conversations every day.

"So, it's Valentine's Day," she says. "The food triggers are everywhere; it's all chocolate; it's all my favorite stuff. And no one is going to buy *me* flowers; he just left for *her* . . . My boss started talking about reorganization, focus, and streamlining . . . There's all this cold, wet stuff coming down out of the sky . . . I think I'm getting a cold . . . Maybe I have some other vicious disease . . . I feel old and creepy and all I want to do is give up . . . What now, Theresa?"

"What a nasty place to be in," I say to my client. "What will help you?"

Then, I explain that now is not the time to answer the phone call from your ex-mother-in-law or from that woman at work you can't stand. Instead, sit down, have a good cry, and wrap yourself in your favorite blanket. Let yourself feel bad. When you're done, wipe your eyes, blow your nose, and get out your journal or a pad of paper because you're going to create a list . . .

> ### EXERCISE: What now

1. Answer the question: What can I do?

    *No, it's not the time to strangle your ex-mother-in-law. It's too cold and wet out there. But put it on the list anyway. Calling your boss or sending a nasty email won't work either—neither will the "I'm disappointed" email.

2. List the changes that could make you happy.
3. Now list what you really, really want and need in your life.
4. Decide what your next step will be.

Reading Food Labels

Get in the habit of reading food labels before you buy or eat the food. This is important. So important that I tell my clients, "If you are unwilling or unable to read the label on a food product, please do not buy it or eat it until the food label is available."

Get in the habit of reading food labels before you buy or eat the food.

The front of the label is where the manufacturer presents the product in the best possible light; the back of the label, in the Nutrition Facts box and the Ingredients List, is where the truth resides. Ingredients are listed in decreasing order by weight. When looking at breakfast cereal, the order in which ingredients are listed becomes important. If sugar is the first ingredient, that means there is more sugar than any other food in the product.

If you are sensitive to sugar, you want it to be as far down the ingredient list as possible. Again, everyone is different. Some can tolerate foods that have sugar listed as the third ingredient; many can tolerate foods that have sugar listed as the fifth ingredient; others the eighth ingredient; some cannot tolerate foods that have sugar listed at all. I suggest you start with the fifth ingredient and see how that works. But this is your recovery; do what you think will work best for you.

Be wary when there are several different sugars in the ingredient list; if they were all added together, sugar might become the first or second ingredient. Often, you can easily choose a lower sugar product just by reading the label. Tomato products especially vary widely, both by brand and by product, in the kinds and amounts of sugar they use. Salad dressings also vary widely, and there are many excellent tasting salad dressings now available with no sugar and no artificial sweeteners.

And, as I've mentioned before, take sugar from all the foods that aren't important to you. I'm guessing you will find plenty of these.

One day, I sent my husband to the grocery store to buy hamburger. We were having a barbecue, so he brought home prepared hamburgers—which is fine, except the label said beef, dextrose, and salt. The dietitian said to her husband, "We don't need sugar in our hamburgers!" So, back to the grocery store he went: "Could you please tell me why you need to put sugar in these hamburgers?" he asked. "Well, I'm not really sure, sir," she said; then she took her sugared hamburgers back. He was not happy with me.

The moral of this story is: you will often find sugar where you least expect it. I can tell you categorically that you do not need dextrose in your hamburgers. You can add water (water does not always have to be declared on the label). But a mixture of sugar, water, and salt will make the hamburger hold together much better; it will also make it weigh more so they can charge hamburger prices for sugar water. They may also believe that if it's sweet and tastes good, you'll buy more.

You'll find details about food labels in a bonus lesson, which you can access here: www.sanefoods.com/bonus.

Weighing and Measuring

The Sane Food Solution's food plans are created and designed to meet your body's nutrient needs, to take away your drug and trigger foods, to balance your body's blood sugar and neurochemicals, and to give you comfort and confidence about your food and eating. When the food plan clearly tells you what and how much you should eat, you can let go of the guilt, the anxiety, and your internal debate over what to eat and what not to eat.

> **When the food plan clearly tells you what and how much you should eat, you can let go of the guilt, the anxiety, and your internal debate over what to eat and what not to eat.**

If you have been eating too much or too little of one of the nutrients, there will be physical, mental, emotional, and spiritual consequences. You may have excess cravings, hunger, sleepiness, anxiety, or irritability. You may feel separated from your feelings or too close to them. To reduce this, establishing a daily practice of measuring and weighing your foods may be the way to go.

Weighing and measuring your food helps in five ways:

1. After weeks, months, or years of abusive eating, weighing and measuring will "recalibrate your eyeballs" and help you see what foods and amounts will work for you.
2. Weighing and measuring give you specific proportions of nutrients; you can see how different proportions affect your well-being.
3. You know what and how much you have eaten; you cannot be vague or deny the truth to yourself. The disease can no longer lie to you.
4. If the food plan does not work for you, you can change it.
5. The food plan helps you disengage your feelings from your eating behavior. Now you can see both more clearly.

There is a lot of resistance to weighing and measuring food; people find it embarrassing, shameful, and annoying. It brings to mind diets and deprivation. Being hungry is not pleasant, nor is feeling deprived or punished about the food and your reasons for taking a different path with it.

But if you're realistic and rational about it, nearly every item bought or sold in the United States is weighed, measured, or counted. The meat sold at the grocery store is weighed when you buy it or when packaged for sale. The chips are in little packages, weighed, and the bag tells the individual weights and the total weight. Your cereal states the serving size, and how much that weighs in ounces and grams. The yogurt is weighed in the container. If you buy cheese or turkey at the deli, they weigh it. All the boxes, from cookies to dish detergent, have weights on them. The pharmacist counts your pills. Outside the grocery store: the gas station measures the gas it puts in your car; the sales associate in the shoe department measures your foot; your doctor measures your heart rate, blood pressure, and cholesterol. You measure the amount of coffee you put in the pot, the amount of water in the rice, the amount of broth you need for soup, and how much chicken is needed for dinner. If you go to a restaurant, someone there can tell you the weights and measures of all the foods they serve. If not, the restaurant will go out of business quickly.

This is not a punishment; it's a practice designed to free you. If you have been struggling with food and eating and diets and weight for a long time, it is possible that your eyeballs may need recalibration.

> **If you have been struggling with food and eating and diets and weight for a long time, it is possible that your eyeballs may need recalibration.**

Your goals are to:

- Weigh and measure your food to get the amounts right to meet your body's needs.
- Never again have to worry about or obsess over having eaten too much or too little food.
- Never again have to struggle so others do not see what you're eating.
- Never again have to feel sick because you ate the wrong food and/or the wrong amounts.
- Clear and sharpen your mind; have your cravings and obsessions fade, your body back to its normal weight; enjoy full, shining hair, smooth skin, strong nails, and lots of energy.

You may not need to weigh and measure forever, or in every situation. But in the beginning, it's important to control portion sizes to be sure you're getting enough and in the right amounts.

If anyone tells you that weighing food is really weird, ignore it. Tell them you're working with a crazy dietitian who thinks you have food allergies, or tell them you're reading this really cool book and following this plan that feels great. (You may not give them your book—let them get their own!) You might ask them why it's important to them or thank them for caring, but you do not wish to discuss it.

Also, you don't need to weigh and measure all foods all your life, unless your addiction makes it necessary. But for the beginning, until we have a plan that works for you, weigh and measure as much as possible to help you get on track.

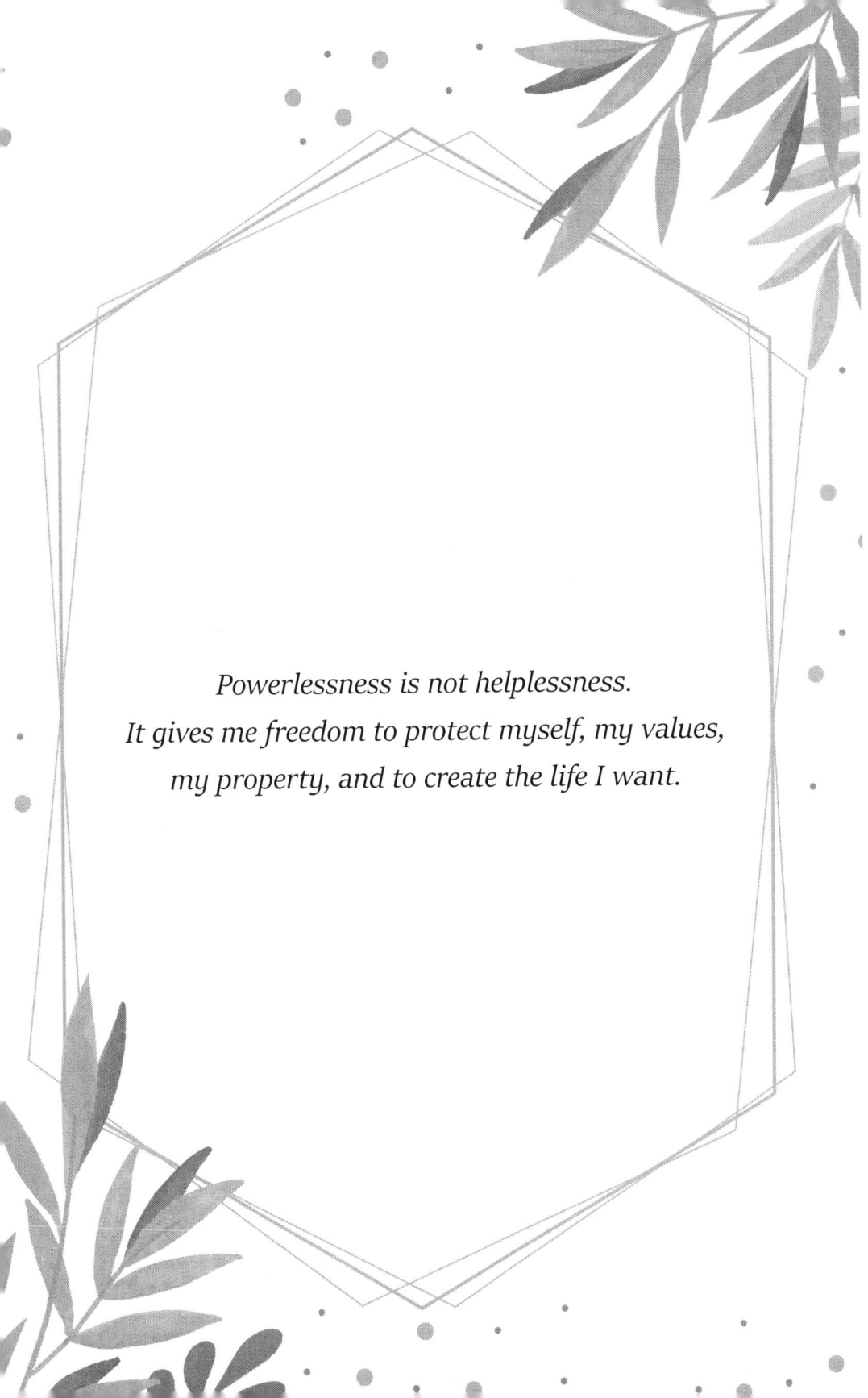

*Powerlessness is not helplessness.
It gives me freedom to protect myself, my values,
my property, and to create the life I want.*

Chapter 10

Support Network

About two years ago, I was teaching a workshop, and I said a sentence, then swallowed my tongue and asked myself if I really believed it. So, I thought about it for years, watched the results of my clients, and now I have decided that I really do believe it to be true. The sentence was this: "Without the help of a Higher Power and other trusted people, I have seen no one recover long-term from addictive eating disorders."

> **Without the help of a Higher Power and other trusted people, I have seen no one recover long-term from addictive eating disorders.**

This is a scary sentence, particularly if you were raised in a dysfunctional and abusive family, like many of my clients. If so, you had to grow up very quickly. You had to learn to take care of yourself because the adults around you were not able to take care of you properly. You may even have found yourself taking care of the adults. You may have found yourself taking care of the other children in the family. Responsibilities that should have been your parents' fell to you, and you did the best job you could. You probably felt lost and alone and maybe even put upon. You hoped that if you did a good enough job, someone would come and rescue you. No one came. The grownups did not "grow up" and take over. You struggled on, alone. You may have reached out for help only to get slapped down with sentences like, "Don't you be telling other people our personal business."

So, you kept quiet and did the best you could.

> **You learned to rely on food to solve your problems or to make the pain go away.**

But food was there. It was your only comfort, your only solace—and it was always dependable. It could be counted on to make the pain stop. You learned to rely on food to solve your problems or to make the pain go away.

Now in recovery, I'm going to ask you to rely on a Higher Power and other people as trusted advisors. I'm going to ask you to say the truth to near strangers, to tell them intimate details, like how you are really feeling. I'm going to ask you to trust your food—your food—to a relative stranger. I'm going to ask you to talk about what happened and to not use your most reliable source of comfort and wholeness to relieve the pain.

==It's going to be really tough. It's also necessary.==

It may seem like I am asking you to break all the rules—both those taught to you and those you created for your own safety. For some people, I am. For others, I am asking you to re-examine the rules, to change some of them, or perhaps to create new ways of being and behaving. This is still hard and scary work.

"Ah, no," you say, "I can do it myself." That's what I was taught, and I used to believe it. It did not work for me. If you find a way to solve this problem without a Higher Power and other people, please come tell me how you did it. We'll start a business, charge a great deal of money to tell other people how to do it by themselves, and within a year we'll close the business multi-millionaires! Funny thing, those who would come to us for answers would violate the very principle.

The moral of the story is people can help. But it takes hard work to get people to help you, to find people who are willing and able to help you, to create a relationship in which they are able to help you effectively. It requires talking to people, getting to know them, letting them know you, and getting to the point of trusting enough to allow them access to the place that hurts.

There are three things I observe in my clients who are unable to create a comfortable, peaceful, abstinent relationship with food and a joyful useful life. The first is the refusal or inability to let go of isolation, to let other people into that "secret private place" that is truly themselves; the second is the refusal to create a relationship with a Higher Power; and the third is the refusal to do the work of transformation known as step work and emotional growth.

The truth is that food served a valuable purpose in your life at one point, and one of the main goals of your recovery program must be to find and create other things that meet your needs as well as or more effectively than food did.

Trusted Advisors

The time has come to set up a strong network of friends and family to support you who will not pull you back into addiction. There are three kinds of trusted advisors to help you through the recovery process. One is the group of other ordinary people who have been working on their eating problem and can help you with yours. The second is the group of professionals you hire to help you. (This group needs to be willing to work together and with the group of ordinary people.) The third is the Higher Power (God or HaShem, for example). Since we've already touched on creating a deeper relationship with your Higher Power in previous chapters, we're going to focus on relationships with other people. And trust.

To trust someone means you feel safe with that person. You feel able to speak the *whole* truth because you believe that person will not think less of you for it. You can rely on that person's care for you—though there may be some covenants, or rules, in the relationships that tell you how things work.

Psychologists call this a "holding environment," where you can feel and heal. You may not feel completely safe because the feelings you need to feel and deal with are the very ones you fear and hate and are most repelled by. So, you need to have enough trusted advisers (a "posse," if you will) that will be broad enough and strong enough to help you over this rocky path to recovery. In this journey, you need friends, confidants, and some professionals. You want wise ones.

One way to know if someone is wise is to look at the results in their own lives. Are they living what the Buddha would call a "skillful life?" "Do you want what they have?" (in the Twelve Step language); "Is Jesus Lord in their life?" (in the fundamental Christian language); "Do you and they see God's movement in their lives?" (in the spiritual language).

> **Remember, how you got into this mess is not how you will get out of it.**

Listen to the advice of those you trust, and trust with care and forethought. Often their suggestions are not what you choose or even feel you can do. But remember, how you got into this mess is not how you will get out of it. You are the one who needs to change your behavior to change your life.

So, how do you find or create your "posse"—and what is a "posse" anyway? Originally, a posse was a group of people called together by the sheriff to help in law enforcement. Here, it means the group of people you trust to help you solve your problems with food and create the life you want.

When it comes to creating your posse, think about our President and his band of trusted advisers. How does he choose them? First, they're people who have experiences in the areas he wants advice on. They are likely to be people who have goals and values like his. They are willing to stand behind the President, to look for and think about the things he needs, and hopefully, to help him see all sides of a situation. They give him advice. And if the advice works the way the President wants, they are likely to be asked for advice again.

Speaking of which, did you know that there once was an "Ex-Presidents Club?" The current President met with the living Ex-Presidents to talk about the issues no one else understands, having never been President. "How did you find time to sleep; when did you find time to exercise?" They may have talked about how hard it was to be retired from the presidency or how it felt to be without that wand of power. Maybe they gave the current President advice about his concerns.

If the current and Ex-Presidents found benefit in talking about their experiences with someone who has been in the same situation, don't you think you might, too?

Now, in private, you may say the truth about the issues to your chosen posse and come to conclusions about what you should try. The biggest blessing of all? Your posse will hold you accountable for your behavior. They will help you look at what worked and what didn't work. And by simply saying the truth in an atmosphere of love and acceptance, you come to see yourself differently and know how to approach your problems. It's truly an amazing feat!

Trusting In Yourself

Before you can trust others, you must trust yourself. As Vicki Carroll puts it:

> The highest form of trust is self-trust. Self-trust is allowing yourself to be who you are and who you were meant to be without fear of reprisal or rejection. It's not taking your hands off the steering wheel and trusting the car to stay between the ditches. It's confidence in knowing that if you keep your hands on the wheel, you can and will safely drive yourself to your destination. It's not an act of submission or omission, but an act of aggression. It requires effort. It's not going with the flow, but it's directing the flow. And with that effort comes the total confidence required to sustain you through your life's difficult times and guide you to your aspirations.
>
> At the same time, self-trust carries with it an element of responsibility. That responsibility is to yourself. If you don't feel it in your gut, know it in your bones, or at least feel like you are progressing toward that end in a relationship, you have an obligation to let go. Otherwise, a cloud of self-doubt will engulf you and destroy what has taken you years to develop—trust in yourself. "To thine own self be true" and thine own self will be trusted. When you trust yourself, you make yourself worthy of the trust of others.[1]

So, the first hurdle is to trust yourself. This will take time—which means you give yourself a break. Give yourself the chance to get to

---

[1] Vicki Carroll, "8 Tips on How to Build Trust in a Relationship," Hub Pages, August 11, 2024, https://discover.hubpages.com/relationships/How-to-Build-Trust-in-a-Relationship.

know you for who and what you really are: which parts do you want to keep, which parts do you want to let go of? It means you're determined, long-term and consistently, to change your relationships with food, yourself, and others. This includes people, your Higher Power, everyone else, maybe even your dog.

You may also need to change your behavior toward yourself. Learn to treat yourself and your body with dignity and respect. This means you no longer speak rudely to yourself or hurt the body with food, or thoughts, or anything else.

It goes back to what we said earlier, acceptance is not approval. You may not trust yourself now because you have seen yourself behave in untrustworthy ways. You may not like the way you behaved. You may choose to change the way you behave. But to trust yourself means to be honest with yourself.

How many times have you told yourself, "I'll have just one," and then eaten the whole bag? You behaved in an untrustworthy way. When you accept that you cannot eat just one, you can begin to be honest with yourself and trust yourself. You'll be able to behave in a way you can trust. (You do *not* have to like it.) Then, you can change your behaviors, change your relationship with those who hurt you, and begin to create the life you really want.

You may find (as I did), the most helpful people are those who know you well enough to say the truth about you and be right. They serve as a mirror for you: who you are, who you want to become, and how to get there.

The Twelve-Step Room

Many people find they have no friends they trust, or the friends

> **You need people who have gone through similar experiences to show you the way through.**

they have do not have the strength or experience to help them with this journey. You need people who have gone through similar experiences to show you the way through. You need folks who understand what you're struggling with and what you're trying to accomplish. Twelve Step programs are very helpful in this: it's a group of people who have been through situations similar to yours, have found the way out, and are willing to talk to you about it.

They can be helpful in providing information, contacts, support, and community. They have a program of recovery that can teach you how to live a different kind of life, to break away from the pendulum swing. Twelve Step programs have clear ground rules and traditions designed to keep you safe and help you learn the process. They have books and pamphlets that help you understand what they and you are about.

Overeaters Anonymous was the first; now there are many groups, each with their own food plans and abstinence requirements; try a few; see what the rules are and what will work for you. What really meets your internal needs is a food plan that works for you, plus a recovery program you can use and trust. But you aren't limited to this program alone. You may wish to utilize Alcoholics Anonymous, Gambler's Anonymous, Workaholics Anonymous, Debtors Anonymous, and many others, even though you don't experience those particular problems. You can test them out by attending an open meeting, which allows outsiders who don't profess to that addiction to participate.

Healing happens naturally in the Twelve Step rooms as you identify with what others say, hear pieces of your own story shared by others, and feel their love and acceptance in your own life. As you listen to their stories, you begin to feel your own feelings and observe them with grown-up, compassionate eyes. As you hear how others resolved these issues (or failed to resolve them), you learn what works and what doesn't work for your problems; you get new insight into how to handle your life and your issues.

Don't give up after one or two meetings; they may seem odd to you, and you may need time to get acquainted. Your first instinct is likely to be to run away, saying it's not for you, or to criticize, saying how sick the people seem or how proud and arrogant they seem about their recoveries. Instead, look for similarities; ignore the differences; find and focus on the positives. See what might work for you. If you still say, "Nothing about this works for me," you'll need to find another group of people you do trust, whose counsel and help do work for you. Rarely have I seen people achieve strong recoveries without a group of people they trust who support them.

Give yourself time to find people who can stand with you in this growth you need to do. Isolation, being alone, not talking about what's going on, is the hallmark of the abusive eating disorder. As much as you may not want to, this is an area you need to confront if you want to be truly well and enjoy long-term recovery.

Find a Sponsor or Two

Within a Twelve Step program, you need to reach out and create a group of friends and advisers; the most common type is a sponsor, who helps you solve your problems with food and create the life you want. No one can do this alone. Let others help you. Let their love and acceptance lead you to the life you want.

Just to clarify, Twelve Step programs are not called "Healthy Persons Anonymous" for some very good reasons: they are open to the public; not everyone there is healthy or trustworthy, and everyone there is in a different stage of recovery. You must pay attention to who you are talking with.

You want to interview people before you appoint them to your posse. Get to know the person. Ask questions: "How did you get started in this program; what was it like for you in the beginning; how has this program helped you; have you worked the steps; what are the steps and why do they help you; what's a sponsor; do you have a sponsor; how do you work with your sponsor; what do you do when you sponsor others; what do you enjoy about the program; what would you like to change about it?"

These kinds of questions will help you understand the person: what you liked or didn't like, if anything said made you feel safe or scared, if you share interests, if the person is someone you'd like as a friend or confidant. Lastly, it helps you answer if the person is someone who's grown in the way you want to grow.

If the answer is no, call a few other people, check out some other meetings, or try a different fellowship. If the answer is yes, check things out some more. Ask more questions. Share a little. Ask directly for confidentiality and privacy. Ask what anonymity means. Tell how you feel about something to see how the person reacts. How does the person handle life: is it skillful; is it how you want to be able to handle it? Do you share and live by the same values? Is the advice right on target for you? Do you feel put down or supported and understood when you talk to this person?

And you may want more than one sponsor. The Debtors Anonymous program has a process I like. Two or three other members are chosen to become your PRG (Pressure Relief Group) and meet with you every few weeks to discuss, support, and set up a recovery plan. This idea may appeal to you. But here is the hardest part—you need to call these folk regularly. You need to meet them at meetings or go share a salad or a glass of iced tea. You need to talk and talk honestly. You need to get to know them and let them get to know you.

To clarify, your sponsors (your posse members) do not need to know each other or communicate with each other, unless there's a situation that warrants it. Think about this for a minute. If you are having a problem—the food is calling you, your mother-in-law is driving you batty, whatever—is it easier to call for help to someone you know well or someone you have spoken to only once or twice? You need to get to know people and create a group of relationships so that when you need a friendly ear, the person you call will be safe and familiar.

The answers to all your problems really are inside you. The problem is that you cannot always see it or hear it by yourself. Your sponsor helps you, listens carefully and lovingly to your words, waits to hear the right answer, then points to it: "There." Now you see your own answer; and it's the right one.

Or perhaps you have a lot of addictive denial. Your sponsor may gently pierce the veil of your denial and help you look beyond it to see your own truth. Often this is done through the telling of stories and how another solved your own problem. This is why Twelve Step meetings and sponsors are so very helpful.

Paid Advisors

There's another group of trusted advisers—those you pay. You may need a physician, a psychiatrist psycho-pharmacologist, a dietitian or nutritionist, a therapist, a physical therapist, a trainer or exercise coach, or a spiritual adviser. These are people you choose to work with on a regular or irregular basis to help with issues in their areas of expertise. Choose carefully.

Ask for recommendations from others in recovery with you, from other professionals you trust, and from your posse. Research and interview professionals before you begin to work with them. Consider their background, certifications (those they have and those they should have, but don't), experience in the field. Do they enjoy working with clients like you; do they offer support groups and classes to help your recovery plan?

More importantly, how do you feel when you visit their office: welcomed, safe? (Do you sense this person knows how to help you or do you need to explain what an eating disorder is; does this person have the same or consistent ideas about recovery as you, believe in the program you want to work, make you feel stronger and more capable; do you feel a sense of positive regard coming from this person to you?)

If your answers are no, move on. Find another adviser. If yes, work with that person on the frequency and time suggested by the advisor. After three months, look at your progress. If you feel stuck, if you feel you aren't making progress or seeing the results you want, if you're struggling with issues that need to be confronted, talk to your health care professional about your concerns. Get to the bottom of the issue.

> **If your paid professional's advice is not working for you, don't keep doing the same thing for ten years.**

If your paid professional's advice is not working for you, don't keep doing the same thing for ten years. Look at what needs to change.

I have been guilty of hanging on to a trusted advisor for too long. A long time ago, I was cleaning out some papers and found one of my journals. I opened it randomly and read a page. "Yes!" I thought. "That's exactly what's wrong and exactly how I feel!" The problem was that page had been written ten years before, and it made me angry. I got up and got to work. I called people till I found someone who could help me effectively and began to work on the solution.

It doesn't make sense to be stuck in the same position.

Paid advisors can also help guard against your own misinterpretations. Again, choose wisely. You won't ask your accountant about your medical condition, but you may want to ask him about the tax implications of taking the time off you need. Likewise, go to your sponsor, therapist, physician for the advice and emotional support needed for you to do what must be done. Listen to their advice and consider it carefully. If you trust them, you should be able to do as they suggest, even if you don't really understand why it would work. Of course, the proof is in the pudding: when all is said and done, it should, indeed, work.

You Are the Boss

You need to surround yourself with people you trust—those who can see your situation from a different vantage point, who can speak truth into your life, who can help you be the person you were meant to be. But even then, you remain the boss.

You can add or subtract people from your support group as you choose—professionals and non-professionals alike.

We discussed the questions you should ask yourself when choosing a professional; when it comes to hiring, you'll want to focus on these three things:

1. Is this person willing to take me in the direction I want to go?
2. Does this person have the right credentials and experience to be able to take me in the direction I want to go?
3. Do I sense that together we can build an alliance, an area of positive regard, so I can feel safe and trusting in the relationship?

If the answer is yes, hire the professional and take the first three sessions to be sure you were right; then go to work: follow instructions, try new behaviors. After three months, look at what you have accomplished. If you find you're not getting the help you need, reevaluate.

The same holds true with your non-professional posse. Create relationships you enjoy. Talk to people about the things that matter to you. Ask for advice. Listen: are their answers about you or them; is their focus on your feelings or their feelings, your struggles or their struggles; do their questions help or confuse you? When you leave their presence, do you feel loved and supported or cold and more alone than before? I dare say, if they aren't for you—if they don't have your back—they shouldn't be a part of your posse.

Keep the advisers you know, love, and trust; add new people, if needed. Then, use them to lead you to the life you have always wanted, to teach you how to learn and grow. Have fun—and return the favor by helping when it's needed.

EXERCISE: Trusted Advisors

Before you set out to create your posse, it's good to know what you're looking for—advisors you may already have in place and those yet to find; what you want and what you do not want:

- Who are the people you trust as much as or more than food?
- What are the kinds of trusted advisers you need?
- What are the qualifications you now have for a trusted adviser?
- What will make you replace a trusted adviser?
- How do you want them to help you?

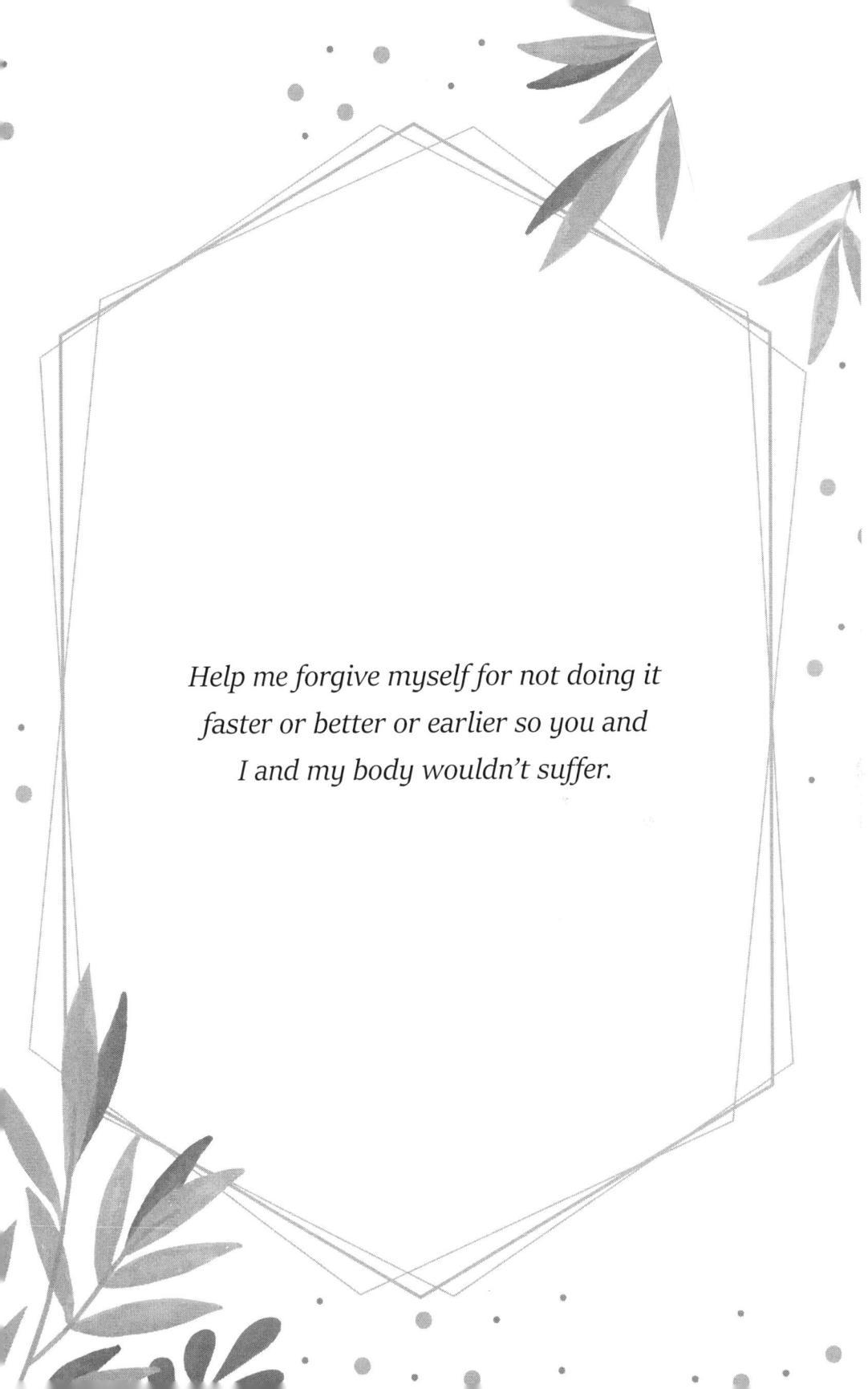

Help me forgive myself for not doing it faster or better or earlier so you and I and my body wouldn't suffer.

Chapter 11

Enjoying a New Life

For some, their body, mind, and spirit react differently to refined and overprocessed foods. This sensitivity becomes an addiction. Food becomes the end all, be all: comfort, reward—even sanity itself. Your addiction to these substances is what has kept you in an endless loop of consumption, malaise, and suppression. The way out is to eliminate foods you can't eat because they throw your brain chemistry off.

Food companies are no help; they have made sure you'll remain addicted to their food. If you don't take these foods out of your system, your body will respond to them. This is not about willpower. This is about learning to eat a whole new way, managing your relationships and your emotions, putting systems in place to avoid temptation because everyday life will place temptations in your path.

There's no such thing as moderation. Until you embrace that, the problem will keep coming back. It doesn't matter what others think; if you don't accept this, you'll yo-yo diet your way through life.

Of course, abstinence is difficult in a world of temptation and unhealthy foods. You need to develop a strategic response to those temptations. You must

> **There's no such thing as moderation.**

cease your feelings of deprivation and reach for peace and freedom. This involves challenging your addictive thinking, banishing the thoughts that hold you down, and learning to use the power of positive thoughts to recreate your world.

As you combat your addiction, you'll learn to treat your body with dignity and respect. You'll nourish it back to health. You'll learn to practice self-care. This is not selfish. Effective self-care helps you create the life you want and helps establish a healthy lifestyle.

Remember, you're "in recovery" from food addiction, so you'll need to create and continue daily practices to support your reclaimed health. Wise boundaries are crucial in this new approach to life. Establish clear guidelines in your relationship with yourself, with food, and with other people. Set up new patterns of attitudes and behaviors that will help you maintain your new lifestyle. And let other people help you because you cannot do this job alone. You can't.

Surrender

"Ooaauugghh! Failure. Despair. Desperation. I'm not good enough; I can't do this. It's too much for me. I have failed again."

Too often, this is how we view surrender. But this is not the surrender I want for you.

Think of it as a good massage: you release your muscles; you let go of your control over them. In return, you feel more relaxed, less pain—over time, you may even find improved flexibility, less anxiety, fewer headaches, better sleep. The massage works. You feel better.

So, it is with surrender . . .

Surrender is your decision; it is not submission.

Surrender is an empowering form of release.

Surrender is an intellectual decision made over time after careful consideration, often in desperation, always with grief. Surrender, and you choose not to fight or control your circumstances, emotions, or situations; you choose to become a willing participant in a different course.

Yes, when you surrender, you give up, but not in the way you may think. You don't give up on yourself or the situation; you give up the notion that you can make reality different than it is.

There is incredible power in that surrender. Strength is found in letting go of a clenched fist and emptying the weight you're holding onto. You release the burden of solving the impossible problem and open yourself to help from others.

> **Release the burden of solving the impossible problem and open yourself to help from others.**

That's right, when you surrender, you choose to accept help; you permit other people and powers greater than yourself to guide you in the right direction. It may be God or your Higher Power that you trust to steer you to a better life, or it may simply be a larger group of people—and their ideas, wisdom, and strategies, different from and more powerful than those you've known—who will help you.

Essentially, when you surrender, you let go of beliefs that are not getting you what you want. It's necessary because it allows you to come to terms with the fact that willpower alone is not enough to solve this problem.

So, surrender . . .

Drop into your body and notice the fear, uncertainty, anxiety that is causing you to want control. Stay with this physical sensation in your body—the energy of uncertainty—that causes you to grasp for control. Be with it fully; allow yourself to feel it. Relax and release it. Walk into your mind and see the feelings, the trauma, the desperation, the hopelessness, the frustration. Let it go. Sweep it out of your mind and let there be space.

Then in the quiet, alone with your true self, make the decision to change your behavior—to feel your feelings and process them, to do what needs to be done to make your life different, to meet your goals, to allow other people and forces to help you, and to reach for the joy, peace, and freedom you have always wanted.

Finally, ask for help. Choose your changes. And begin.

Takeaway Thoughts

As I've said many times before, following the food plan is the first step in the recovery process, and I hope this book has helped you begin to do that.

And while the food plan is the core, the beginning, it is but a step. I want you to get the food far enough out of the way to see and feel and create and enjoy the life you really want to have. When you first put down the abusive food, you'll find you have many difficult feelings. You may be irrationally angry; you may have mood swings, headaches, irritable times, brain fog, and many other uncomfortable feelings. These are likely to resolve themselves if you don't eat over them. They are the symptoms of the body clearing out the accumulated trash and reestablishing itself on firmer ground. It's called withdrawal.

You may feel lost and alone without your abusive foods. Think of this as the "space to create the life

> You may feel lost and alone without your abusive foods. Think of this as the "space to create the life I really want."

I really want." It means you now have choices, first to work a program of recovery that gives you self-care, support, and spirituality, then to begin to restructure your life to be the way you have always wanted it.

Oh, but the peace you will find. These foods to which your body is sensitive have been handling a whole lot of situations that you maybe did not understand or did not know how to deal with. There may be some emotional clearing out you need to do. Oh, but the strength you will find. You will be amazed at your ability to think clearly, make good decisions, and make different choices for your life.

And the skills you will learn: to draw boundaries, answer the questions of others, change how you react to those who used to hurt you, manage those feelings from the past, learn their lessons, and move on.

If you let the Wise Person Within and your newfound Higher Power lead and guide you, if you do the important steps, if you allow other recovering people to help you (and choose them carefully), you will find your emotional and spiritual growth skyrocket. You will be capable of creating a life you never could even have imagined.

May the peace and joy of recovery stay with you always, and may you experience true, full, and long-lasting freedom from the obsession with food. May you be guided by other people and a Higher Power; may you know they believe in you and love you.

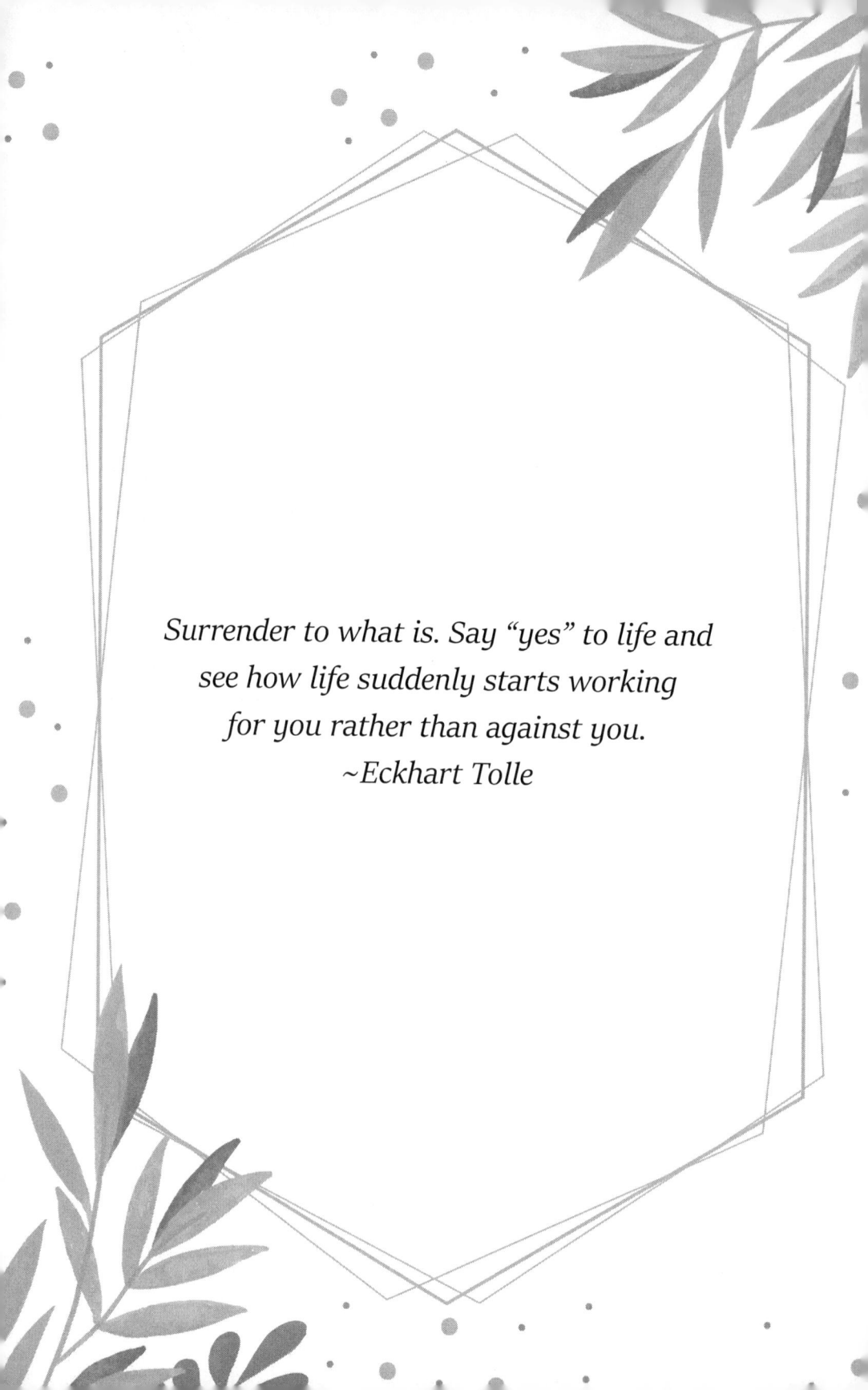

Surrender to what is. Say "yes" to life and see how life suddenly starts working for you rather than against you.
~Eckhart Tolle

A Final Thought

Nothing says radical change quite like the transition from caterpillar to butterfly. Emerging from the state of unchecked food addiction to embracing the sane food solution is no different.

As compulsive eaters, we eat and eat and eat—much like a caterpillar—as if it were our job. We munch on things others wouldn't touch. We hide the evidence of our eating and even of our presence. We avoid predators and feel threatened by many occurrences that others find normal. We try to fit in with the world around us, and we try to be as unobtrusive as possible. We hide when we are scared.

Then there comes a turning point. Sure, a caterpillar may not say aloud, "Something has to change; I'm tired of being a fat lumpy bug." But there's some sort of draw to something better—a call to fulfill a bigger destiny. So, that caterpillar begins to take the steps to transform its body . . . and, eventually, a butterfly is born.

Scientists do not understand the process of how caterpillars transform into butterflies, even though they watch it happen. Similarly, they do not fully understand how and why the recovery process works, even though they can easily observe that it does.

They see that a caterpillar is most vulnerable just as it exits the chrysalis; if it attempts to emerge faster, it could lead to death. And they witness that addicts are most vulnerable in the early stages of recovery. It requires time for recovery "wings" to harden; patience; help from others—but some things can only be done by the one undergoing transformation.

Of course, there are a few differences between a caterpillar's transformation and your transformation:

To start, caterpillars always go for the gold when it comes to daily nutrients. Even if they eat something bad, they make up for it by eating large amounts of nutrient-rich foods: leaves, berries, and plants. In contrast, when you find yourself eating badly, you may be tempted to give up and go back to eating high-calorie, nutrient-free foods. But whatever your recovery stage, when you eat inappropriately, get back on your food plan at the next meal. Eat nutrient-rich foods as often as you are able, consistently, without guilt.

When it comes to the caterpillar's transformation, he goes it alone. The caterpillar seeks out a place of privacy. But if you want to succeed at long-term recovery, do it with the help of other people: therapists, nutritionists, sponsors, physicians, other helping professionals and non-professionals, and especially other suffering people. In general, they will be different people than those you relied upon when you were eating foods you are allergic to. You need new attitudes and a different kind of direction to create this transformation. You need people who can support and guide you.

Caterpillars make their transformation in ten to twelve days. For you, it could take years of hard work. Don't give up. It's worth the wait.

There is also a price to pay for becoming a butterfly. Namely, there's no going back. The chrysalis doesn't beckon the butterfly; the butterfly is not tempted to go back to the life of a caterpillar. Yet you can easily go back to compulsory eating.

A FINAL THOUGHT

In your mission to stay on track, you can learn a thing or two from the butterfly:

Butterflies seek out nectar to fuel their flight. You should be the same, on the constant lookout for the right nutrients to fuel your mind and body.

Butterflies stay focused on the goal. If a butterfly gets off course on the way to California or Mexico, it takes a short time to reorient itself before heading in the right direction yet again. "Stay the course" should be your mantra, as well. Whatever distracts, whatever diverts, you need to reorient yourself to the direction you want to go as soon as you can.

Butterflies avoid predators by diversion and confusion; they remove themselves from dangerous situations. You need to do the same. Learn how to recognize and protect yourself from folk who threaten your abstinence. Then, become skilled at diversion; avoid situations that threaten your abstinence.

Butterflies view the world through ultraviolet and polarized light, meaning they can see colors and patterns undetected by the human eye. Similarly, you need to learn to see differently—to begin to view the world with a recovery lens. Recovery needs to change your perspective, your priorities, and indeed, your whole life.

Male butterflies also go mud puddling—it's a way to absorb minerals and salts for later "fun." Yes, recovering is hard—there may even be ugly aspects of it. But don't forget to have fun. It gives you strength to be who you need to be for the rest of your life.

And if conditions are too cold, butterflies find a safe, warm place to shelter until conditions improve. If they're in captivity, they may be placed in plastic containers with food and water. There will be times when you need to find a place of refuge, and there will be times when you need help getting to that safe place.

May you learn the wisdom of the butterfly. May you allow yourself to be present in each moment, to flutter and float with joy and freedom, to be part of the beauty of the universe. May you enjoy each sip of nectar, each sunny day, each moment of being alive.

Blessings to you,

Theresa

Appendix

Withdrawal Symptoms

Physical Symptoms	Day	Mental/Emotional Symptoms
	1	
	2	
Headaches; Diarrhea alternating with constipation Hunger	3	
	4	Strong food cravings
	5	
	6	
	7	
	8	Anxiety
	9	Irritability
	10	Mood swings
Fatigue Nausea Body aches	11	Strong food cravings
	12	
	13	
	14	
	15	
	16	"Fuzz brain" alternating with Periods of clarity of mind
	17	
	18	
	19	Rage
	20	

Profound fatigue "Like walking through knee deep peanut butter"	21	"Fuzz brain" alternating with Periods of clarity of mind
	22	
	23	
	24	
Chest congestion Coughing	25	
	26	
	27	
	28	
Fatigue continues	29	
	30	Periods of clarity of mind lengthen
	31	

Recommended Resources

Thank you for reading *The Sane Food Solution*, which includes tools and strategies other chronic dieters have used to free themselves from abusive eating once and for all. To support your continued progress, you may find the following resources useful.

Your Personal Food Plan Guide

Your Personal Food Plan Guide is a sane, easy-to-use, gentle guide to creating a food plan that really works for you. Discover a food plan system for recovery from food addictions, from all addictive and compulsive eating behaviors, and from sensitivities to refined, processed, and man-made foods. It is sugar- and flour-free; wheat and other allergens are indicated.

Find information from the latest nutritional research on topics such as celiac disease, wheat vs. other flours, and beans, nuts, seeds, and lentils.

Delicious Recovery I, II, and III

Each of these cookbooks includes basic recipes for breakfast, lunch, and dinner including salads, vegetables, and starches; main entrees and mixed dishes; even safe muffins. All recipes are sugar- and flour-free and already adjusted for your food plan. These recipe collections include foods you can feed your family and your guests without difficulty. Foods to enjoy!

Visit Sanefood.com/products
to purchase these cookbooks, and more.

Get Your Free Bonus Material

As an additional thank you for reading this book, I've created a special section of checklists and mini tutorials that **never made it into the book!**

>FREE< Visit
Sanefood.com/bonus
to get your free bonus materials.

About the Author

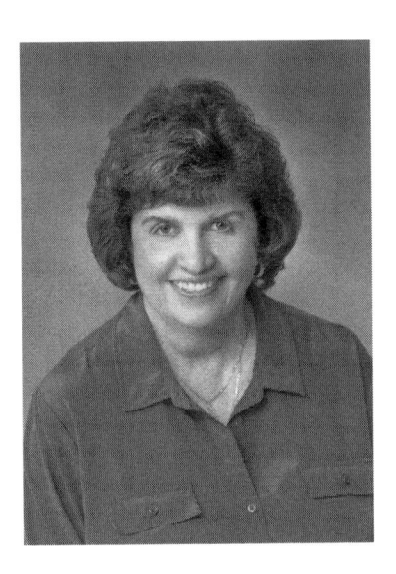

THERESA WRIGHT, RD, is a dietitian and nutritionist, and a pioneer in the burgeoning field of food addiction. Nationally recognized for her innovative approach to nutrition and the treatment of weight issues, Theresa was among the first nutrition experts to recognize untreated food addiction as the reason millions of people struggle with food and weight.

As founder of Renaissance Nutrition Center, Inc., Theresa has developed a ground-breaking recovery program aimed at healing self-destructive eating behaviors. Changing lives for nearly thirty-five years, the program uses a gentle, sensible, and evidence-based approach that is tailored to fit each client's unique needs.

Theresa Wright is also a sought-after speaker at conferences, workshops, and retreats. She provides programs and consulting services for corporations, treatment facilities, and professional organizations.

She co-wrote the chapter on food addition, "From the Front Lines," for the first comprehensive collection of academic literature on food addiction. (*Food and Addiction: A Comprehensive Handbook*, edited by Kelly Brownell and Mark S. Gold).

In addition to writing for professional publications, Theresa writes for lay audiences, as well, including her revolutionary food plan, *Your Personal Food Plan Guide*, and three volumes of cookbooks, *Delicious Recovery*.

Theresa Wright has been named one of Today's Dietitian magazine's "10 Incredible Registered Dietitians Who Are Making a Difference." And because of her expertise in treating addictive and compulsive eating disorders, she was invited to be a contributing consultant to the Overeaters Anonymous food plan guide, *Dignity of Choice*. She also wrote a chapter for the Appendix of *The Beloved Brown Book*.

Theresa Wright holds B.S. and M.S. degrees in Nutrition Science from Drexel University, is a Registered Dietitian and a Licensed Dietitian-Nutritionist and has been awarded a Clinical Supervisor by the European Certification Board.

See her website at www.sanefood.com/.